Avian Medicine and Surgery

LIBRARY OF VETERINARY PRACTICE

LIBRARY OF VETERINARY PRACTICE

Avian Medicine and Surgery

B.H. COLES BVSc, MRCVS

Distributed in the USA and Canada by
BLACKWELL/YEAR BOOK MEDICAL PUBLISHERS • INC.

BLACKWELL SCIENTIFIC PUBLICATIONS
OXFORD LONDON EDINBURGH
BOSTON PALO ALTO MELBOURNE

© 1985 by
Blackwell Scientific Publications
Editorial offices:
Osney Mead, Oxford, OX2 OEL
8 John Street, London, WC1N 2ES
23 Ainslie Place, Edinburgh, EH3
  6AJ
52 Beacon Street, Boston
  Massachusetts 02108, USA
667 Lytton Avenue, Palo Alto
  California 94301, USA
107 Barry Street, Carlton
  Victoria 3053, Australia

First published 1985

Set by Text Processing,
Clonmel, Eire

DISTRIBUTORS

USA
  Blackwell Mosby Book Distributors
  11830 Westline Industrial Drive
  St Louis, Missouri 63141

Canada
  The C.V. Mosby Company
  5240 Finch Avenue East
  Scarborough, Ontario

Australia
  Blackwell Scientific Publications
  (Australia) Pty Ltd
  107 Barry Street
  Carlton, Victoria 3053

British Library
Cataloguing in Publication Data

Coles, Brian H.
   Avian medicine and surgery—
   (Library of veterinary practice)
   1. Birds—Diseases
   I. Title
   636.089'6   SF994

   ISBN 0-632-01403-2

Printed and bound in Great Britain
by Butler & Tanner Ltd,
Frome and London

Contents

Preface

There is an increasing public interest in birds. More people are keeping aviaries and ornamental waterfowl. Membership of bird-watching societies is increasing. Falconry has seen a considerable revival, and conservation groups are encouraging captive breeding of wild species for re-stocking.

For these reasons veterinarians in practice are increasingly being consulted on avian problems. Apart from some instruction in the specialized field of poultry science, the veterinary graduate receives little or no formal instruction in the medicine and surgery of general avian species.

The purpose of this handbook is to give some guidance to the busy general practitioner presented with a medical or surgical problem concerning birds, with which he may not be very familiar. The book may also be of some value to those undergraduates who feel that this area of veterinary science has not been adequately covered during their training.

A volume of this size cannot pretend to be comprehensive and it is inevitable that it will not be detailed or specific enough on certain subjects. It is assumed that the reader will have a basic knowledge of the anatomy and physiology of the domestic fowl.

The various diseases are not dealt with in the more usual academic method by organ systems, but rather in the form of principal diagnostic signs as presented to the clinician. In this form it is hoped that the handbook will be more readily usable by the veterinary practitioner.

I should like to thank all those colleagues who, by referring their clinical cases to me and by discussing their avian problems, have expanded my knowledge of disease in birds.

I am grateful to Professor A.S. King for advice regarding some aspects of respiratory physiology in the chapter on anaesthesia. My thanks go to Dr John Baker who read Chapters 2 and 3 and gave valuable advice. My thanks also to Miss Underwood who read and gave helpful advice on Chapters 4, 5 and 9. I am particularly grateful to Ted Chandler for reading and editing the whole book and for his continual encouragement. My thanks go to Jane Ratcliffe for permission to print the schedule of bird releases obtained from her meticulously kept records. I thank the editor and publishers of the *Journal of Small Animal Practice* for permission to print large sections of my paper on 'Nursing birds'. Also I thank the editor, the authors and publishers of the *Journal of Anatomy* for permission to adapt the diagram used here as Fig. 3.1. My thanks to the publishers of *Veterinary Clinics of North America* for permission to use Table 2.1.

I am grateful to Mrs. J. Padmore and to Mrs. S. Postlethwaite for sharing the typing and for helpful criticism of the manuscript. Finally my thanks go to my wife, Daphne, for showing considerable patience and constant encouragement during this task.

Brian H. Coles.

1 / Clinical Examination

History

Before starting to examine the bird in detail it is important to obtain from the owner as much information as possible. Particular attention should be paid to the following questions:
* What has the owner noticed wrong with the bird? Falconers will often notice a change in a hawk's performance which may be an early sign of disease.
* Are there any other birds kept by the owner and have any of them been ill or died?
* Has the owner bought in any other birds recently?
* How long has the patient been in the owner's possession?
* Has the bird been ill before and has it had any treatment?
* Have there been any changes in the environment which may have put it under stress? Some individuals within a species are more highly strung and therefore more easily distressed than others.
* Has the owner changed the food or bought in a new supply?
* In the case of raptors, was the food fresh? If the food was stored in a deep-freeze was it properly defrosted? Falconers feed their hawks with meat from a canvas bag. This should have a separate, easily cleaned plastic lining. Some falconers become careless and the meat becomes contaminated from a dirty bag. Ask if the droppings (called mutes by falconers) have changed in character.

Other relevant questions will occur to the experienced clinician and the answers should be sought from the client. However, owners vary greatly in their powers of observation and the practitioner may find it rewarding to hospitalize the avian patient so that a more accurate observation can be carried out.

Examination of the cage or surroundings

The character of the droppings

Always try to examine some fresh droppings. When the client makes the initial inquiry on the telephone tell them not to clean the cage out before coming to the surgery.

The cloacal excreta usually consist of a dark-coloured central part

1

(from the rectum) and an offwhite-coloured surrounding portion consisting mainly of urate crystals from the kidneys. The consistency and to some extent the colour of the droppings vary with the species and the diet of the bird. Fruit eaters, such as mynahs and starlings, have rather fluid droppings. Even parrots, which normally feed on a seed diet, will develop more fluid droppings if fed with a lot of fruit. On the other hand, geese have a more bulky and rather more formed stool. It is therefore important that the practitioner is familiar with what is normal for each species.

As to be expected in birds with an enteritis, the dark, central part of the droppings becomes more fluid; the reverse is true in constipation. However, in birds that are not feeding or that are feeding inadequately the central part of the droppings tends to be of a watery, greenish nature. Birds with pancreatic disease show excessive droppings that are buff grey in colour and waxy in texture. Test these for starch with Lugol's iodine. Excessive or decreased urate crystals indicate a renal problem. Undigested seed or grit in the droppings is always abnormal and indicates a malfunction of the gizzard. Blood in the droppings may come from the rectum, the cloaca or the oviduct. This may indicate ulceration, possibly involving a neoplasm. Sharp foreign bodies, such as pieces of metal, can be ingested and can reach the rectum in some birds such as ducks.

Blood in the cage

Blood spattered round the cage may have come from the cloacal orifice or it may be from an injury to the wings, feet, beak or body. If the blood is widely spread, it is probably from wing trauma, possibly a damaged growing feather.

Regurgitation

With small birds, examine the cage bars, perches, mirrors and other cage furniture for any evidence of adherent small flecks of white material. This may be evidence of regurgitation. Regurgitation is normal courtship behaviour in the male budgerigar. The young are fed in this manner also. However, this normal behaviour can develop into a pathological neurosis and the bird will sometimes even attempt to feed its owner.

Raptors daily produce pellets or castings formed in the gizzard composed of the undigested parts of the diet (skeletal tissues, feathers, fur, etc.). The colour of the castings will depend on the diet but they should be of a crumbly, almost dry texture and have no offensive smell. Liquid or putty-like castings or those with blood or excessive mucous are abnormal. Many other species of birds such as thrushes (Turdidae), crows (Corvidae) and herons (Ardeidae) normally produce pellets.

Other observations to be made on the cage

In the case of seed-eating birds, note whether the seed is being dehusked or simply being scooped out of the feeding dish and onto the floor.

In the case of psittacines note whether the perches or any of the toys are being chewed. The clinician should also observe if there is any sign of rust on the cage structure and see if the paper on the floor of the cage is being chewed.

With a magnifying lens it may be possible to see signs of parasitic mites on the cage fittings. These appear as minute black, red, orange or greyish-white specks, which are seen to move. Mites hide in cracks and crevices and emerge to feed on the bird at night, so they are best seen with a torch in a dark room or when the electric light is switched on suddenly.

Observation of the patient

If an experienced aviculturalist or falconer brings you a bird and says that it is ill, even if you cannot see anything abnormal, the chances are that the bird has something wrong with it. The changes that take place in a bird from one that is completely healthy to one in the early stages of illness are so subtle that it takes an experienced observer to notice them. The problem with most sick birds is that usually by the time someone realizes that they are ill, they are very ill. The bird should have a full-rounded, bright eye, with no sign of the membrana nictitans. An eye which is slightly oval means that the bird is not fully alert. Any bird that spends all its time huddled in the bottom of the cage, taking no notice of an observer, is near death.

The plumage of the bird should be sleek and lie flat over the body. If all the body feathers are ruffled, the bird is trying to conserve heat loss.

Breathing abnormalities

A bird that is obviously dypsnoeic with its mouth open and gasping, may not necessarily have a respiratory condition, but is certainly very ill. Tail bobbing in small birds is a sign of an impaired respiratory system also. In both these types of abnormal breathing, a space-occupying lesion of the abdomen may prevent the full expansion and contraction of the posterior air sacs, so that air flow through the lungs is considerably reduced. Cyanosis is sometimes indicated by a blue colouration of the beak and legs. If the part of the neck in the region of the crop slightly inflates with each expiration but breathing is otherwise normal, this may indicate some obstruction of the outlet ostia of the anterior air sacs where these connect with the secondary bronchi. A change in the voice, which becomes more harsh, or a change in pitch in the sound from a raptor could indicate a problem with the syrinx. Hypovitaminosis A with or without secondary bacterial infection and abscessation involving the tissues of the syrinx could be responsible for these signs. Falconers talk of 'kecks' and 'snits' (sneezing) in their birds. An incessant and often irritating high-pitched squeak in the budgerigar is sometimes due to pressure of the enlarged thyroid on the syrinx. This is initiated by an iodine deficiency and a consequent hypothyroidism. Clicking or asthmatical noises, which may be almost imperceptible unless carefully listened for, can be caused by viral, bacterial, fungal or yeast infection of the respiratory tract or by the nematode, *Syngamus trachea*, which affects many species of birds. In the latter case, obstruction of the airflow in the trachea is enough to cause gaping typical of the disease.

A change of voice in a bird always indicates a pathological condition of the syrinx and therefore prognosis is much more serious. This contrasts with the situation in the mammal where a change in voice indicates an upper respiratory condition and the outlook is more favourable.

Central nervous system signs

Birds may show any of the following signs: torticollis, opisthotonus, ataxia, circling, paralysis and clonic spasms or fits. All these may be caused by deficiency of B or E vitamins, infectious disease, poisoning, concussion, cerebral vascular disturbances and tumours.

It is not uncommon for a budgerigar to be presented with the acute onset of a variety of the above signs. Making a specific diagnosis is difficult and the prognosis is always grave. Thrombosis is said by Hasholt (1969) to be uncommon in birds, but atheromata are recorded from a range of species. Hasholt (1969) records the cases of arteriosclerosis of the carotid arteries in three old amazon parrots. This was believed to have resulted in cerebral ischaemia because the birds kept falling off their perches.

In diurnal raptors hypocalcaemia and hypoglycaemia are both common causes of fits. Most important among the infectious diseases causing nervous signs is *Newcastle disease,* which affects all species. The variant of this organism, *Paramyxovirus,* causes nervous signs in pigeons both domestic and feral.

A rhythmic swinging of the head from side to side, particularly in owls, is indicative of vestibular disease and is equivalent to nystagmus in mammals. A flaccid paralysis with an inability to hold the neck up ('limber neck') is seen in botulism and lead poisoning, particularly in swans but also in other birds (Borland, Morgan & Smith,1977). Folic acid deficiency can also cause paralysis of the neck in turkey poults.

Wing injuries

A dropped wing may be due to nerve paralysis but is most likely to be due to injury to the bones or muscles. Some idea of the part of the wing that is damaged can be gained from observing exactly how the wing is held. If the injury lies between the digits and the middle of the radius and ulna, the primary feathers are usually trailing on the ground (Fig. 1.1 a). Injury to the elbow or the humerus very often results in the

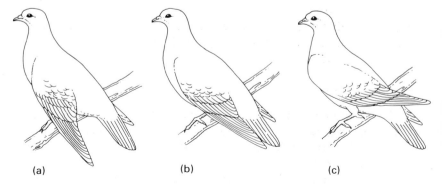

(a)   (b)   (c)

Fig. 1.1. How the wing is held after injury to different parts of the skeleton.

wing being held lower than that on the normal side but the primary feathers are held up off the floor (Fig. 1.1 b). Injury to the coracoid or shoulder joint causes the wing to be rotated so that, although the whole wing is lower, the primaries are above the level of those on the opposing side (Fig. 1.1 c).

Since there is considerable interspecies variation in the relative lengths of the different sections of the wing and, consequently, variation in the weight of these parts, the signs will not only depend on the nature of the injury (bone, muscle or nerve) but on the species of bird involved. Small birds in particular may sustain quite serious fractures of the wing bones and still look quite normal. An accurate diagnosis can only be made by a detailed inspection and possibly by radiography.

Handling birds

Before attempting this in the case of a small and obviously sick bird, it is wise to warn the owner that there is a risk that the bird may suddenly die of heart failure when an attempt is made to catch it. This can occur with apparently healthy birds not used to being handled.

To reduce this risk, the task can be carried out in a dark room using the light from a torch covered with a red filter. In many cases it is then possible to pick the bird straight from its perch. However, some birds see better in subdued light than others.

When handling the larger birds care should be taken to control the feet of raptors, which have a powerful grip, and also to watch the beaks of the larger parrots which can cause a severe biting injury. Small raptors can strike out rapidly with their feet. A hawk which is hooded is often easier to handle, although some falconers are reluctant to use a hood. Hooding any bird of prey (trained or wild) usually has a sedating effect and the use of a towel or even the cut corner of a large brown paper envelope placed over the head is quite effective.

Birds such as herons (Ardeidae), storks (Ciconiidae), rails (Rallidae), gulls (Laridae) and gannets (Sulidae) can use their beaks as stabbing weapons. Cormorants (Phalacrocoracidae) can attack with the hooked end of the beak.

In all these cases a strong pair of welders or industrial gloves is invaluable. Tamed raptors and parrots can be handled without gloves if the bird is used to being handled, but the clinician would be well advised not to take any chances.

All the large birds are best cast on a cushion or soft surface before examination. The wings need to be held gently but firmly to the body with no undue pressure placed on the thorax.

Physical examination of the restrained bird

In a bird that is not too ill, the clinician might find it easier to carry out a more thorough examination if the bird is under moderately deep sedation or light anaesthesia. Refer to the section on anaesthesia.

Feathers and plumage

The plumage should be of a good, even, dense colour. Barbules should lock together so that the feathering gives a uniform outline to the body form. In the normal bird only the axillae are sparsely covered in feathers. If the areas of skin covering the lumbo-sacral and sternal regions are thinly covered or are covered in an abnormal greyish fluff instead of the usual contour feathers, the cause may be of nutritional or endocrine origin, e.g. thyroid. Progressive feather loss with a typical white, flaky, but thickened skin may be due to ringworm (*Trichophyton* spp.) infection, particularly if this is seen around the head and neck. In poultry a zinc deficiency has caused dermatitis and failure of feather growth. Sometimes, particularly in parrots, there may be evidence of self trauma. In this case, apart from skin wounds, the vane of the flight feathers may be chewed or the shaft may be crushed (as distinct from snapped or broken off). Some of the growing feathers may have been plucked leaving bleeding follicles. Plucked feathers are usually replaced quickly and new feathers can be seen emerging. Examine these new feathers to see if they are short and club-shaped. See if they have a circumferential constriction or are curled or deformed. Any of these signs may indicate a viral infection or nutrient deficiency. Self-mutilation may be due to frustration or boredom or stress brought on by a change in routine or initiated by over-preening during the breeding season. It may be initiated by parasitic infection. Mite infestation may lead to invasion of the feather follicle and damage and loss of the feather. Both mites and lice can cause irritation. A careful search of the plumage will show any lice situated along the feather shaft or on the skin surface. Healthy birds groom themselves to keep infestation in check, sick birds do not. Examination of the skin or of the powdery remains of a feather shaft with a magnifying lens will be necessary to identify any mites present. Feather picking by an incompatible or dominant cage mate is not uncommon. This may be worse during the breeding season.

Malformed and curled flight feathers or those without proper vane formation are usually the result of faulty nutrition (inadequate essential amino acids or vitamin deficiency), but may also be the result of chewing by lice or other infection. In parrots the yellowing of green feathers may be due to a deficiency of the amino acid lysine. Feathers that are frayed or have the shaft cleanly broken or snapped off are the result of careless handling or inadequate caging. In the budgerigar and some other psitticines the condition called french moult, in which fledglings lose some of their primary wing and tail feathers, has been given a number of causes. It has been said to be due to infection of the feather follicles due to poor hygiene, to early and intense breeding or to excessive vitamin A intake. The condition, in fact, may be multifactorial. Some recent work by Pass & Perry (1984) indicates this may be part of a syndrome which affects many psittacine species and which may be viral in origin. The minute structure of feathers may be permanently damaged after contamination with mineral oil, even after this has been completely removed. The barbules may not hook together properly. Lines of decreased density and weakness across the vane of the feather, known variously as 'fret', 'hunger' or 'stress' marks, are recognized by falconers but are also seen in other birds. These are believed to be caused by a check in growth of the proliferating cells of the epidermal papilla during the formation of the feather in its follicle and may be accompanied by other feather defects. Moulting or feather replacement takes place in most birds at well defined intervals,—once, twice or three times a year. In a few species such as cranes and eagles moulting may be every two years. However, in parrots the process is continuous. Nutritional or infectious conditions that cause feather abnormalities often have similar effects on the germinative cells of the beak and claws.

Occasionally a developing feather will fail to emerge properly from the feather sheath. The folicle continues to enlarge pushing its way below the surface of the skin and a feather cyst is formed—a condition most commonly seen in canaries but also seen in other breeds. The cyst is often associated with an inflammatory condition of the skin and causes marked irritation to the bird, so that the bird picks at the cyst and may rupture it.

The head region

After detailed examination of the plumage it is best to continue with an examination of the head region starting with the eye.

The eye

The observer may see a variety of conditions. Keratitis, oedema of the eyelids and blepharospasm due to a foreign body are relatively common. Matting of the feathers around the eye can be evidence of epiphora which may be unilateral or bilateral. If bilateral, this could be due to lesions blocking the opening of the naso-lacrimal ducts, where they are situated close together in the posterior part of the choanal opening. Swellings just above or below the eye may be evidence of sinusitis of the supraorbital and infraorbital sinuses which may have progressed to abscessation. Brown, crusty eruptions around the eyelids and commissures of the beak may be due to avian pox. In budgerigars the powdery white encrustations of cnemidocoptic mange mite infestation may extend from the cere to the areas around the eye and the commissures of the beak. This may also be seen in other species. Retrobulbar neoplasms of the orbit and tumours of the nictitating membrane have been recorded. Examination of the anterior chamber of the eye may reveal evidence of hypopyon, or hyphaema, or damage of the iris. Fluorescein should be instilled onto the surface of the cornea to detect any scars or ulcers. All these lesions are not uncommon, particularly in owls, and may be due to fighting or to road traffic accidents.

Examination of the eye reflexes is generally difficult but is somewhat easier in raptors, because of the proportionately larger-sized eyes. The pupillary light response is difficult to elicit, because the muscle of the iris is striated and partially under voluntary control. It is also affected by emotional disturbance of the bird. A rapid pupillary light reflex indicates central blindness because conscious control may have been removed due to damage to the brain. Pupils may be widely dilated after concussion resulting from an accident. Consensual pupillary light reflexes do not take place in birds because all optic nerve fibres completely cross over at the optic chiasma and representation on the cortex of the optic tectum is contralateral. Touching the cornea produces a pupillary response and a consensual response is shown in the other eye. If a bird is not too frightened, it will sometimes show a fixation reflex towards an interesting object.This can be shown by using food (for a raptor) or a glittering object (for a corvid) moved from side to side in front of the eyes.

A blink reflex of the eyelids or nictitating membrane reflex may be stimulated by a threatening gesture. This should preferably be carried out from behind a transparent screen.

Cataracts are not uncommon and can be seen with or sometimes without an ophthalmoscope. Examination of the posterior chamber with the ophthalmascope is less rewarding. There is no reflective tapetum in birds. The optic disc is obscured by the large vascular projectory of the choroid, known as the pecten. The shape and size of this structure varies in the different species. The retina appears as a uniform granular tissue usually grey or brownish red in colour. Hyper-reflectivity and synchisis scintillans is reported by Greenwood & Barnett (1980) in a wild tawny owl.

For a more detailed discussion of the functional normality of the avian eye the reader should refer to the chapter by Greenwood & Barnett (1980) in the reference section.

The ear

This is not obvious in birds since there is no pinna. In most birds the external orifice is covered by modified contour feathers. In owls the ears are large and placed asymetrically, a condition which improves directional sensitivity. Because of its nearness to the eye, the ear may be involved in trauma affecting the eye. Attention is drawn to otitis externa by the feathers being matted around the external ear. Small (1969) reports the protrusion of the tympanic membrane through the external orifice but this is a rare condition.

The skin of the head

This should be examined for any sign of subcutaneous haemorrhage due to accidents or wounds that may be caused by fighting.

The cere and external nares

Look for any discharges which may vary from catarrhal to dried exudate. Nasal exudate is often due to hypovitaminosis A and superimposed microbial infection. Staining of the feathers above the cere is evidence of nasal discharge. This may be blood stained. Excess growth of the cornified tissue of the cere, a condition often seen in budgerigars and called brown hypertrophy is of no clinical significance unless the nares become blocked (Fig. 1.2).

In the male pigeon (Columbidae) there may be a similar exuberant growth of the cere. In the budgerigar, the cere is pink in the immature bird, blue in the male and brown or buff-coloured in the female. Birds that show some blue and brown colouring may be intersexes with both one ovary and one testes present in the abdomen. Reversal of colour may indicate chronic illness.

Knemidocoptic mange infection is not uncommon in budgerigars and can affect other psittacines as well as other species. It is shown by a greyish, scabby, crumbling texture of the cere often accompanied by excrescences around the commissures of the beak and the eye. The burrowing tracts of the mite can sometimes be seen in the horn of the beak. Diagnosis can be confirmed by scraping the lesion. After clearing the scrapings with 10% potassium hydroxide, examine under a microscope. Trauma to the cere can be the result of a collision during flight or from a caged bird flying at the mesh work of its cage. Damage to this area may involve the cranial facial hinge situated between the premaxilla, nasal and frontal bones. Occasionally a neoplasm may involve this region.

The beak

Examine the beak for any evidence of cracking or splitting, which may be a sign of underlying fractures of the premaxilla or mandible. Care should be taken when examining some birds such as gannets and some

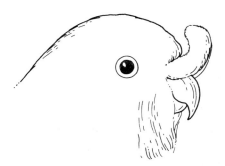

Fig. 1.2 Brown hypertrophy of the cere.

ducks in which the edges of the beaks are quite sharp. Toucans (Ramphastidae) and mergansers (*Mergus*) have a serrated edge to the beak. Cracking of the horny beak may be traumatic or a sign of vitamin A deficiency or infection. Overgrowth or distortion of the beak may be due to a neoplasma (e.g. osteosarcoma) or trauma to the proliferating epidermal cells or due to knemidocoptic mite infection. Deficiency of vitamin D, calcium, biotin and B vitamins are all said to cause abnormal beak formation (Altman, 1982). Raptors fed on an artificial diet that does not need very much tearing of the food before swallowing, can develop a marked overgrowth of the upper beak. Parrots can develop beak abnormalities brought about by wear on their cage bars by constant climbing. The beak is a constantly growing and changing structure. Some wild birds, e.g. oystercatchers (Haematopodidae) have a comparatively rapid growing beak which can develop a different shape adapting the beak to different feeding habitats. Those feeding on cockles develop a spatulate shaped beak, whilst those feeding on earthworms develop a more pointed beak.

The mouth and oropharynx

In aquatic birds a piece of fishing line protruding from the pharynx may be attached to a fish hook embedded lower down the alimentary canal. Diagnosis can be confirmed by X-ray or by endoscope. Fish hooks may damage other birds and the author has even seen one case in a blackbird (*Turdus merula*).

To examine the mouth of a conscious powerful bird some sort of speculum may be necessary. A pair of artery forceps can be placed between the two beaks and then opened, or the speculum of a canine auroscope can be utilized.

There is considerable interspecies variation both in the anatomy and mobility of the avian tongue. The typical parrot has a blunt piston-like tongue whilst that of the woodpecker (Picidae) is very long and mobile. For more detail the reader should refer to the publication by King & McLelland (1979). Abscesses are seen sometimes on the surface of the tongue and small pin-point lesions of candidiasis may be observed also. Both these conditions may be brought on by vitamin A deficiency. This leads to a hyperkeratosis of the epithelium of the mucus-secreting glands (Gordon & Jordon, 1977; Jones, 1979). Abscesses may also be seen anywhere on the mucus membranes of the mouth, particularly around the choanae where they may block the naso-lacrimal opening. Closer inspection of the nasal mucus membrane can be carried out by endoscope examination through the choanal space. Abscesses in the mouth may be bacterial in origin or they may be the early signs of trichomoniasis. This is seen more usually as an extensive cheese-like diptheritic membrane covering the oropharynx and sides of the mouth. This disease occurs in a number of species but is particularly common in pigeons (Columbidae) when it is called 'canker' by pigeon owners and has also been known for many years by falconers to occur in raptors, when it is called 'frounce'. Again, hypovitaminosis A may predispose to this condition. The lesions of both trichomoniasis and candidiasis look very similar and may occasionally be confused with capillaria infection.

Avian pox lesions may be seen at the commisures of the beak, in all species particularly in passeriformes, columbiformes, raptors and psittacines. However, they are not seen in galliformes or anseriformes.

The glottis is a slit like opening into the larynx and trachea lying on the floor of the mouth usually just posterior to the root of the tongue. In some species such as herons (Ardidae) it lies farther back. Neoplasms and exudative lesions can affect this area resulting in partial obstruction of the airways. Sinusitis of the infraorbital sinuses can lead to a gross swelling, filled with catarrhal exudate, on both sides of the oropharynx. This condition can be caused by mycoplasma and has been seen in a number of species including parrots (psittacines), gulls (Laridae), mynah birds (Gracula) and raptors. Cooper (1978) advocates digital examination of the mouth and oropharynx and laboratory exploration of any exudate obtained.

The neck

This should be palpated for any swelling which may indicate a foreign body impacted in the oesophagus (e.g. a bone wedged in a raptor's throat) or an impaction of the crop, which can occur in most species. A fluid swelling may be due to the condition of 'sour crop', when there may be excessive gas present also. The crop in the budgerigar may swell also due to thyroid enlargement obstructing the organ. This is sometimes accompanied by regurgitation. Neoplasia of the thyroid, although rare, may be responsible for similar symptoms (Blackmore, 1982).

Many seed eating birds temporarily store seed in the crop but this should not feel hard to the touch. Gulls (Laridae), penguins

(Sphenisciformes) and cormorants (Phalacrocoracidae) store food in the oesophagus and can easily regurgitate this food.

Examination of the body

After the thoracic inlet at the base of the neck has been examined, the clavical and coracoid bones should be palpated for evidence of fractures. In the latter case observe how the wing is held when the bird is free standing [Fig. 1.1 (c)]. Skin wounds around the thoracic inlet are commonly seen in pigeons (Columbidae) as a result of collision with telegraph wires during flight. They sometimes involve the crop and associated air sacs. Subcutaneous emphysema around the thorax may indicate a ruptured air sac, particularly rupture of the cervical or interclavicular air sacs. Rupured air sacs often resolve spontaneously.

The condition of the pectoral muscles should be assessed by palpation. They should be symmetrical but one side may be found to have undergone atrophy, in which case the bird's flying ability will be affected. The condition of the pectoral muscles is an important guide to the overall nutritional state of the bird. The carina of the sternum can be felt but should not be very prominent. Decubitus of this region is common in heavy birds such as geese and swans that are unable to walk. Accumulation of fat and lipomas are common over this region of the pet budgerigar.

The ribs and scapulae should be carefully palpated for fractures. Auscultation of the lateral thorax or at the thoracic inlet may reveal abnormal sounds, though it may be difficult to pinpoint these. Heart murmurs are sometimes detectable in the larger birds. Cooper (1978) describes some cardiovascular conditions encountered in raptors at post-mortem.

The region of the thoracic vertebrae and the syncrosacrum

These areas should be carefully examined for wounds caused by predators or fighting amongst cage mates. The preen (or uropygial) gland should be examined for impaction or neoplastic changes.

The abdomen

In the larger birds it may just possible to palpate the tip of the liver beyond the edge of the sternum. Should the liver be easily felt it is probably enlarged. This can be confirmed by radiography.

The ease with which the abdominal contents can be palpated will obviously depend on the size of the bird. In birds smaller than a budgerigar this is almost impossible to carry out safely without putting too much pressure on the air sacs. In some species, e.g. auks (Alcidae), there is very little room between the sternum and the pelvic bones. However, even in budgerigars it is possible to distinguish a fairly large, rather irregular neoplasm from a regular, smooth and rounded retained egg in the female. The female often has a history of laying several eggs, then has suddenly stopped and the bird is often noticeably unwell. Occasionally a solitary egg may form and cause obstruction.

In slightly larger birds (e.g. pigeons—*Columba livia*) the thick-walled gizzard is easily palpated as firm and globular with angular margins and its retained grit can be felt to grate between the fingers.

In raptors the full or impacted stomach can be distinguished as a rather fusiform softer-walled structure.

Softer and more fluid enlargements of the abdomen which can become quite pendulant in the perching bird, sometimes without apparent ill effect, may be due to either ascites or rupure of the abdominal muscles. Ascites can be confirmed by very careful paracentesis. This is carried out in the midline at the most pendulant part of the swelling. The ascites is often due to neoplasia of the liver or gonads. In female birds, a soft abdominal swelling may be due to an enlarged oviduct caused by salpingitis. Contrast radiography can help in the differential diagnosis. This may be accompanied by an egg peritonitis and a noticeable illness.

Large cyst-like swellings over the abdomen can be differentiated from true ruptures by radiography. The cloaca should be palpated. It may contain a calculus of impacted urate crystals or show a prolapse. Cooper (1978) recommends digital exploration of the cloaca in the larger bird, with a well-lubricated, gloved finger and microscopical examination of the evacuations. An auriscope speculum inserted into the emptied cloaca can sometimes be helpful to examine the mucosa. Matting of the feathers around the cloaca together with excoriation of the surrounding skin can indicate either an alimentary or urinary problem. If the adherent mass is mainly composed of faecal material, then the problem is probably due to diarrhoea. If the concretions are white, and especially if this is accompanied by an impacted cloaca, then the bird has a kidney problem. Since the urodeum is the posterior part of the cloaca in which the urates from the kidney and ureters collect, any impaction in this region due to a urate calculus will necessarily hold up the evacuation of faecal matter in the anterior part of the cloaca or coprodeum and the bird will become constipated. Paralysis and prolapse of the penis may occur in some ducks where two or more male ducks are kept together. This is due to bullying and damage to the nerve supply (Humphreys, P.N., 1984; personal communication).

The body temperature of a bird can be taken via the cloaca, but since there is such a great interspecific variation as well as a normal diurnal variation in individuals, this is not especially helpful in clinical examination. The body temperature of most birds falls within the range $40 - 42°C$.

The wings

Examine each wing bone separately for any evidence of fractures, or luxations of the joints. Excessive mobility of the shoulder joint compared with the other side, together with a wing that is slightly dropped at the shoulder could indicate a rupture of the tendon of supracoracoid muscle (deep pectoral) which can be only confirmed by surgical exploration. Swellings of the bones may be due to old fractures or to tumours or infections. In pigeons (Columbidae) swellings and suppuration of the joints may be due to salmonella causing a chronic arthrosynovitis (Gordon & Jordon, 1977). In raptors injury to the carpal joints may result in a bursitis (called 'blain' by falconers).

In young birds, deformation of the bones may indicate metabolic bone disease due to calcium/phospherous imbalance in the diet.

Waterfowl fed on a diet too high in protein (over 18%) can develop an outward rotation of the carpal joint ('slipped wing')—the primary feathers are relatively too heavy, because they grow faster than minerals can be laid down in the bone.

The mobility of all joints should be checked and compared in the two wings. Comparison should be made of the swelling and development of the muscles for signs of atrophy. Examine the propatagial membranes, which stretch between the shoulder and carpal joints and form the leading edge of the wing when this is fully extended. These are often damaged in flight and may show evidence of scar tissue formation. This results in the wing not being fully extensible or the proximal attachment of the membrane being displaced more posteriorly. In both cases the bird's flying capability may be affected. However, some birds can still fly, but they veer off to the normal side.

Feather cysts and neoplasms are commonly found in the carpal area. They are not always easy to differentiate except by biopsy and/or surgical incision. Tumours in this area are easily damaged and may bleed profusely.

The legs and feet

Each of the bones of the leg should be examined for any evidence of fractures or luxations. This may be difficult with the femur in small birds or in such birds as auks (Alcidae) where this bone is well covered by muscle and dense feathering.

In fledgling raptors the tarso-metatarsal bones are inwardly rotated in a 'hand-holding' position. As the bird grows and begins to take weight on its legs, the feet rotate outwardly to the normal position. In some young birds with metabolic bone disease this does not happen and the gastrocnemius tendon becomes permanently displaced medially. The bird becomes a cripple. In some artificially reared waterfowl fed on a too high protein ration (i.e. over 18%) the Achilles tendon can also become displaced. The bird grows too fast and becomes too heavy for the rate at which calcium and phosphorus can be incorporated into the bone of the leg. A similar condition called perosis occurs in poultry and has been seen in parrots, (Smith, 1979). This is caused by manganese deficiency. This mineral activates several enzymes required for the formation of chondroitin sulphate concerned in bone growth (Butler & Laursen-Jones, 1977). The scales of the legs should be examined for any evidence of swelling, ulceration or scars caused by excoriation of identification rings. In the budgerigar swelling due to a tight ring can become suddenly an acute problem—restriction to the blood supply to the foot can lead to ischaemic necrosis or gangrene. The feet should be examined for any evidence of abscesses. This condition, known as 'bumblefoot', is seen in cranes, penguins, waterfowl, domestic fowl and especially in raptors; the heavier birds are at greater risk. Bumblefoot abscesses may extend as far as the hock and may erode the bones of the foot. This can be confirmed by a radiograph. Smaller birds such as budgerigars may show abscesses on the feet that may be difficult to distinguish from the tophi of gout due to accumulations of urate crystals.

If the suspected tophi are opened and the contents placed on a slide, confirmation that urates are present can be attained from the following test: the crystals are mixed with a drop of concentrated nitric acid and carefully evaporated to dryness over a Bunsen burner. A drop of ammonia is then added. If urates are present a mauve colour will develop.

Knemidocoptic mange mite infestation can occur on the legs of many Passeriformes, particularly Crossbills (*Laxia curvirostra*) and causes the nails to slough. In canaries the condition has long been called 'tassle foot' (Fig. 1.3). Although the infection is common on the

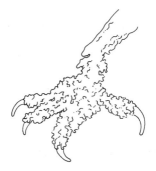

Fig. 1.3. 'Tassle foot' as seen typically in canaries.

head of budgerigars it is not often seen on the feet. In Passeriformes the lesions on the legs can be confused with avian pox lesions and papillomas. Claws that are overgrown through 'tassle foot' and other causes can easily become broken and bleed. Frostbite has been reported in a number of raptor species and in some aviary birds through clinging to frost-covered wire mesh.

2 / Aids to Diagnosis

Simple laboratory investigations

Collection of blood samples

There are three main sources from which avian blood samples can be obtained: the claw, the jugular vein and the brachial vein. The last of these three sites is illustrated in Fig. 2.1, and is probably the easiest place from which to gather enough blood for clinical purposes. Usually a 25-gauge $\frac{5}{8}$-inch hypodermic needle is found to be satisfactory for collection. Because of the fragile nature of avian veins, haematoma formation often occurs and pressure should be applied with a swab as soon as the needle is withdrawn. In the larger birds where restraining the wings is a problem, the right jugular vein can be used. The left jugular is much smaller in most species of birds. When using either the brachial or jugular veins, it may be necessary to pluck first a few feathers to see the vein, after which the area can be cleansed in the normal way. When blood is collected from a claw, the claw needs to be cut with nail clippers from top to bottom, as illustrated in

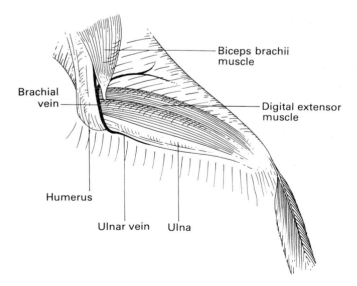

Fig. 2.1. The position of the wing veins used for venipuncture.

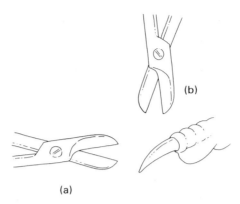

Fig. 2.2. Clipping the claw for collection of a blood sample. (a) This is the correct way to clip the claw for collection of a blood sample. (b) This tends to compress the blood vessel.

Fig. 2.2. Cutting the claw from side to side tends to compress the blood vessels and blood does not flow so freely. After clipping the claw the adjacent, soft tissues of the toe often need to be alternatively squeezed and released to obtain sufficient blood. After obtaining a blood sample from the claw, bleeding should be stopped by pressure from a swab, or if necessary, by cauterisation using a silver nitrate pencil.

A method of collecting blood from the medial metatarsal vein in ducks, first described by Murdock & Lewis (1964), can be used in some other species. When collecting blood, particularly from small birds it should not be forgotten that the circulating avian blood volume can be anything from 6 ml to 10 ml per 100 g live weight. Accordingly, in a 40 g budgerigar the circulating blood volume may be as little as 2.5 – 3.0 ml. Six drops of blood is approximately 0.3 ml which represents 10% of this circulating blood volume. Consequently, if one is not to produce a state of shock in a small bird, 0.5 ml is the maximum quantity of blood which should be taken from a bird the size of a budgerigar. In the average-sized amazon parrot 2 ml of blood can be obtained with safety.

Haematology

The haematocrit or packed cell volume (PCV)

By using microhaematocrit heparinized centrifuge capillary tubes, determination of PCV is quick and easy. The result provides valuable information. In most birds normal values for PCV can be 40 – 55%. More precise details are given in standard texts such as those edited by Petrak (1982), Fowler (1978) and Harrison (1984). After determination of the PCV the serum can be drawn off with a micro pipette and used for obtaining biochemical information.

Blood smears

Only one drop of blood is needed for a smear that can provide information on blood parasites and a differential white cell count. Slides can be stained with Leishman's, Wright's or Giemsa stain. However, avian blood does need a somewhat longer staining period than mammalian blood, at least 5 minutes, and the buffered water used for washing the slide after staining needs to be more acid, pH 5 instead of pH 7, and should be left on the slide for at least 5 minutes. Avian white cells can be more difficult to find than the corresponding mammalian cells. Apart from the fact that the avian red cell is nucleated, the leucocytes in the blood smear are scattered throughout the slide and not aggregated at the edges of the smear as in the case of mammals. There is also much more variation in the appearance of leucocytes in avian blood. Unless a practitioner is carrying out a lot of avian work, it is probably better to fix the slide with methanol and send it to a specialist laboratory for examination. A very useful reference to basic avian haematology is that by Campbell & Dein (1984).

Total red and white cell counts and haemoglobin values

All these values can be obtained by using standard techniques. The figures for a number of species is given in the standard texts edited by Petrak (1982), Fowler (1978) and Wallack & Boever (1983). As a guide, the values for total red cell counts range from 2.5 to 4.5 million mm³ with a mean value of 3.5 million mm³. The figures for haemoglobin vary from 11 to 19 g per 100 ml of blood.

In general there is a wide range of values for different species of birds. The smallest birds with the higher metabolic rate tend to have higher values for red blood cells (RBCs) and haemoglobin. There is also a variation depending on age and seasonal activity. Values for wild birds tend to be higher in the seasons of migratory activity and when birds are flying at high altitudes and low oxygen tension.

The counting of white cells is made more difficult because the nucleated avian red cells cannot be selectively lysed to make counting of the white cells easy. As with the differential white cell count, the total white cell count is better carried out by a specialist laboratory.

Clinical biochemical information

The simplest value to be determined and one which is a useful prognostic guide is total serum protein. For small birds one drop of serum, obtained after carrying out a PCV in a microhaematocrit, can be placed in a hand-held refractometer. Normal values range from 5.2 to 2.5 g/dl, with a mean value of 3.8 g/dl. A value below 2.3 g/dl indicates a poor prognosis for the avian patient. Other serum chemistry profiles have been obtained for some species and are contained in standard texts such as that edited by Fowler (1978). As a guide, see Table 2.1.

Microbiological investigations

Since bacteria and fungi take an important part in the development of avian disease, the clinician should try to establish what potential pathogens are present. However, it is easy to make a hurried decision and conclude that some innocent micro-organism is the sole cause of the disease process.

Birds pick up a variety of micro-organisms from their contacts such as wild birds, rodents and human handlers. Birds newly introduced into an aviary can bring in disease. The United Kingdom insists at present that recently-imported birds undergo a 35-day quarantine period, but this is only to protect national poultry flocks against Newcastle disease. Other diseases such as chlamydiasis (psittacosis), salmonellosis, avian tuberculosis or Pacheco's parrot disease can be introduced at the same time. Also cage and aviary hygiene can sometimes leave much to be desired, and perches, food and water containers become contaminated.

Bacteriological swabs can be taken from a variety of sites such as bumblefoot abscesses, suspected cysts, wounds and natural orifices including the trachea. They can also be taken after paracentesis of abdominal fluid. In the first instance they should be cultured on blood agar plates at 37°C and the organism checked for antibiotic sensitivity.

Faecal swabs are best obtained direct from the cloaca, the vent

Table 2.1. Avian clinical serum chemistries. By permission of the publishers, reprinted from the *Veterinary Clinics of North America*, **13** (2) (May 1973), edited by R. B. Altman DVM.

Determination	Mean	Range
Total bilirubin (mg per 100 ml)	0.23	0.07 – 0.39
Direct bilirubin (mg per 100 ml)	0.15	0.03 – 0.27
Indirect bilirubin (mg per 100 ml)	0.07	0.01 – 0.15
Urea nitrogen (mg per 100 ml)	4.0	2.8 – 5.2
Cholesterol, total (mg per 100 ml)	163	122.4 – 203.6
Alkaline phosphatase (milliunits per 100 ml)	80.3	62.1 – 98.5
Total protein (g per 100 ml)	3.1	2.66 – 3.54
Albumin (g per 100 ml)	1.7	3.3 – 2.1
Globulin (g per 100 ml)	1.4	1.1 – 1.7
A:G ratio	1.3:1	0.78 – 1.82:1
SGOT (Reitman-Frankel units per/ml)	210	193 – 227
SGPT (Reitman-Frankel units per/ml)	44	36 – 52
Thymol [turbidity (units)]	1.93	0.37 – 3.49
Sodium (mg per 100 ml)	110	none
Calcium (mg per 100 ml)	8.3	7.3 – 9.6
Chloride (mg per 100 ml)	109	100 – 122
Glucose (mg per 100 ml)	265	161 – 360
Uric acid (mg per 100 ml)	6.7	2.2 – 7.2
Phosphorus (mg per 100 ml)	3.8	1.6 – 6.1

having first been cleaned and sterilized with a quaternary ammonium antiseptic. If this is not possible the swab can be taken from faecal droppings on a clean surface. When a bird is first handled it will often eject fresh faecal matter from the proctodeum and this can be utilized. A useful method of collecting uncontaminated faeces from small cage birds is to substitute the sand sheet in the bottom of the cage with a piece of X-ray film. Faecal swabs should be routinely cultured on blood agar and MacConkey agar plates.

When *Salmonellae* are suspected, enriched culture media will be needed and culture is best carried out by a specialist laboratory. *Salmonellae* are found in most species of wild birds and easily spread to aviary birds by faecal contamination. However, *Salmonellae* do not appear to be common in the faeces of raptors (Needham, 1981). *Salmonella typhimurium* is by far the most common specific organism in this group isolated from birds.

It should be noted that a wide variety of bacteria are normal commensals in the gut of many birds and these may be pathogenic only if the bird is subjected to stress. A careful assessment of the patient is necessary before one can be reasonably certain that the organism isolated is causing the disease. To some extent the spectrum of avian gut flora is influenced by the diet of the bird. *Escherichia coli* is a normal inhabitant of the gut of most raptors and is probably acquired from the intestine of the prey species. (Needham, 1981). Gram-negative bacteria are not normally present in large numbers in the alimentary tract of grain and fruit eating birds but may become more evident when the bird starts eating insects during the breeding season.

Trachael swabs can be taken in the anaesthetized or sedated bird and a human naso-pharygeal calcium alginate swab is very useful for this purpose.

When *Aspergillus* is suspected, swabs should be cultured on Sabouraud's dextrose agar at 37°C for 36 to 48 hours. Redig (1981) describes the use of air-sac washings in the investigation of respiratory disease. These are obtained by inserting a sterile, flexible catheter, attached to a syringe into the last intercostal space of the bird, and injecting 3 ml of sterile saline (in a large bird 3 kg and above) and then immediately withdrawing this fluid for culture.

Swabs should be taken from any eggs that have failed to hatch. The surface of the egg should be first sterilized with alcohol before a small hole is made in the shell and a swab used to sample the contents.

Swabs should be cultured on blood agar and MacConkey agar, because faecal contamination is a common cause of infection of the egg. (Refer to Chapter 8, p. 189).

When taking swabs from post-mortem specimens, one should take into account that cultures obtained from birds that have been dead more than 24 hours may not be representative. Some organisms, such as *Proteus,* that are normally present in the gut of some birds (e.g. raptors) may rapidly invade other organs after death and overgrow other pathogens on a culture plate.

Examination of stained smears

This is quick, and although not conclusive, it is a useful guide to examine stained smears of pus, faeces and exudate. These can be stained with Gram's stain, methylene blue (for bipolar staining of *Pasteurella*), or where *Avian tuberculosis* is suspected with Ziehl-Neelsen stain. Liver impressions smears can also be stained for acid-fast organisms. Where *Chlamydia* (psittacosis) infection is suspected these smears can be stained by a modified Ziehl-Neelsen technique to show up the intracytoplasmic inclusion bodies. The modified Ziehl-Neelsen technique is carried out as follows: the slide is flooded with dilute carbolfuchsine stain for 10 minutes but is not heated as in normal Ziehl-Neelsen staining. The slide is then washed and decolourized with 0.5% acetic acid—not acid alcohol which is normally used. Decolourization is carried out only for 20 to 30 seconds until the slide is very faintly pink. Counterstain with methylene blue in the normal manner. The tissue cells may then be seen to contain clusters of very small red intracytoplasmic inclusion bodies. However, because of the risk of zoonotic infection, investigation of this disease is best left to specialized laboratories that have the necessary air extraction safety cabinets.

Woerpel & Rosskopf (1984) state that it is generally considered that the presence of Gram-negative bacteria is abnormal in caged birds. Routine staining of a sample by Gram's method can help in the interpretation of antibiotic sensitivity testing. The stain will indicate the relative numbers and morphology of Gram-negative and Gram-positive bacteria and also if yeasts are present. This technique may show anaerobic bacteria to be present when there is little or no growth with a routine blood agar culture.

If *Aspergillus* is suspected in a post-mortem preparation, a portion of the lesion can be teased out on a slide and treated with 20% KOH. The alkali clears the other tissues and renders the fungal hyphae more easily seen. If necessary they can be subsequently gently washed, fixed with heat and stained with lacto-phenol cotton blue. Suspected lesions of *Candida* can be stained with Gram's stain or mixed with Indian ink or nigrosin stain, when the budding yeast like cells may be seen. *Candida* can also be stained with lacto-phenol cotton blue stain.

Diagnostic cytology

Examination of samples taken from a variety of sites and obtained at the same time as those for bacteriology can be a useful aid to diagnosis. Samples for cytology can be obtained by direct contact impression smears or by making a smear of a deposit or fluid sample, in the same way that blood smears are made. The smear can then be stained with Wright's stain or Giemsa stain or fixed in the conventional manner and stained with more selective stains. A good description of this technique is given by Campbell (1984).

Biopsy

Biopsy specimens can be most easily taken from surface neoplasms. They may also help in the diagnosis of skin lesions such as those caused by avian pox virus when the typical inclusion bodies may be found. Biopsies may be taken also from internal organs under direct vision via a laparoscope. An ingenious technique for lung biopsy was described by Redig (1977). A 25-gauge needle is inserted through the penultimate intercostal space into the lung. Tissue is sucked out by syringe and the contents ejected onto a slide for tissue staining. Histology of post-mortem tissues may be necessary to confirm a diagnosis of such disease as Pacheco's parrot disease. This often shows few signs except slight mottling of the liver and the typical acidophilic intranuclear inclusion bodies in the liver cells and sometimes the kidney cells.

Examination of faeces for evidence of helminth infection

Birds carry a variety of helminth parasites. Many birds kept in outside aviaries will easily become infected from the faeces of wild birds which may shed large numbers of parasite eggs. Imported birds may be carrying unfamiliar parasites from their country of origin. Faecal samples should therefore be examined on a routine basis. If the first sample is negative, subsequent samples on alternative days should be examined as some species of helminth parasites shed their eggs intermittently. Also, if the owner has recently but inconclusively wormed his birds, then samples are best not examined for several days as some drugs, especially if used at sub-optimal doses, merely supress egg-laying rather than completely kill the parasites. Faecal samples can be examined by the standard flotation and centrifugation concentrating techniques.

Laparoscopy

Laparoscopy in one form or another has been used in man and animals since the early part of the twentieth century. However, only recently during the last decade, with the development of the human arthroscope, has the technique been applied to birds. It was first used in birds to determine the sex of those species that do not show sexual dimorphism—the so called technique of surgical sexing. Other methods of sexing birds are discussed in Chapter 8, p. 180. However, apart from the direct visual inspection of the avian gonads, it is also possible to evaluate the state of many of the other organs. It is possible to see much of the kidneys, the adrenal glands, the posterior surface of the lungs, the heart, the liver, the proventriculus, the gizzard and the intestines. It is also easy to see parts of the air sac system. Laparoscopy is therefore a useful tool to aid in the diagnosis of many conditions.

The equipment

The endoscopes used for this operation have been designed for the inspection of human joint spaces and range in diameter from 1.7 mm to 2.7 mm. A larger 5 mm instrument can be used on larger birds or sometimes even in birds down to 200 g in weight, when it is necessary to do photography. The apparatus consists of a light source, a flexible light guide and the arthroscope, together with a trocar and cannula. The latest systems now use a fluid-filled light guide. The endoscope is made up of an outer bundle of glass fibres, transmitting light into the organ being viewed, which are wrapped around an inner core of lenses forming the viewing telescope. The whole is encased in a stainless-steel sheath. The angle of vision varies with different instruments from direct-forward to retrograde. The direct-forward viewing lens is the simplest to use for avian laparoscopy.

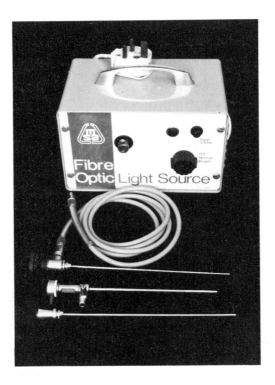

Fig. 2.3. The essential equipment to carry out laparoscopy. The light source, the light guide attached to the 2.7 mm arthroscope, the cannula and the trocar.

Operative methods

Various entry sites to the bird's body are favoured by different authorities for viewing the gonads and other organs. The author prefers the technique demonstrated to him by Samour (1984). The anaesthetized bird is placed in right lateral recumbency with the left side uppermost. The left leg is then drawn forward and held in this position by an assistant or by a restraining tape. In birds below 400 g in weight it is often easier if the operator holds the left leg and left wing out of the way of the incision site. The area of the incision is found in the angle formed just posterior to the proximal end of the femur and anterior to the pubic bones [Fig. 2.4(a)]. Methods used by other operators are to pull the left leg posteriorly and to make the incision midway into the space between the anterior edge of the femur and the

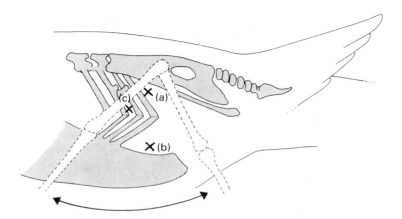

Fig. 2.4. Entry points (a), (b), (c) for laparoscopy in relation to the skeleton.

last rib. Bush (1980) describes using the sternal notch, a landmark in the angle formed between the sternum and where this is joined by the last rib [Fig. 2.4(b)]. Böttcher (1980) makes his incision between the last two ribs just above the angulation [Fig. 2.4(c)]. Whichever point of entry is used, it is very important, particularly in small birds, to get the bird correctly positioned and to be certain of the anatomical landmarks. Before use, the instrument is sterilized using either ethylene oxide gas or by cold sterilization with benzalkonium chloride (1:2,500) or gluteraldehyde solution (Full strength with 2% active ingredient). The latter method is more convenient when a number of consecutive surgical sexings are being carried out. After cold sterilization the endoscope is rinsed in sterile water and dried with a sterile towel. Together with the endoscope it is necessary to have a scalpel fitted with a number 11 blade and useful to have a selection of sterile ophthalmic instruments available.

The operation can be carried out using either a general or local anaesthetic. Local anaesthetic is only really suitable for a quick inspection of the gonads, when a large number of surgical sexings are being carried out consecutively. General anaesthesia allows much easier and safer control of the patient, with much less risk of damage to internal organs by the endoscope. In addition there is more time to carry out a thorough inspection of all viscera.

Having correctly positioned the anaesthetized bird, the operation site is plucked free of feathers. Only the minimum number of feathers necessary to clear the area should be removed. The region is then cleaned and sterilized with a quaternary ammonium antiseptic, taking care not to get the bird too wet. An alcoholic or iodine preparation can be used to complete the process. The operation site is then draped with a transparent plastic or paper drape. Both of these are lighter in weight than cloth drapes and a transparent drape enables the bird's respiratory rate to be seen during the operation. Either type should contain a small central opening.

A small incision 4 – 7 mm in length is made and any bleeding from the skin vessels is controlled because this is liable to cloud the distal end of the endoscope during insertion and obstruct the view. Also any subsequent leak of air from the air sacs during expiration will cause blood on the surface of the skin to foam and obscure the incision. The cannula, fitted with the trocar, is next inserted through the underlying muscle using controlled pressure and at the same time slightly rotating the trocar backwards and forwards. To minimize trauma and reach the desired area it is most important to aim the trocar and cannula in the right direction. If the site using the angle between the femur and pubic bone is used, the instrument is directed downwards and forwards at a slight angle to the vertical away from the vertebrae so that it is travelling more or less towards the centre of the abdominal cavity. In the other methods the trocar and cannula are directed vertically in a direction parallel to the plane of the thoracic and lumbar vertebrae. If the procedure is carried out correctly, the operator can feel the slight pressure on the trocar suddenly 'give' as it pops through the muscle layer into the abdominal cavity. The trocar is then withdrawn leaving the cannula in position so that the arthroscope can be inserted. Should there be any blood on the trocar when this is withdrawn, the whole operation is stopped immediately. During manipulation of these instruments it is best to be seated and to have the elbows resting on the table. The left hand supports the cannula near the point of entry and the right hand controls and directs the trocar and laparoscope. This position of the operator allows delicate and careful control of the instruments. In small birds below 60 g and down to 20 g in weight, the arthroscope can be inserted after the initial incision has been made in the muscle, by pushing a pair of mosquito artery forceps into the incision and opening these slightly to expand the incision. Care must be taken not to bend or break the arthroscope when applying this method.

Problems associated with the technique

No method is without hazard. The first site of entry described has the slight risk that the sciatic nerve and femoral blood vessels may be damaged. In all methods if care is not taken and the instrument is pushed in with too much force or is wrongly directed the viscera could be damaged. Obviously rupture of the heart or of a main blood vessel will prove rapidly fatal. However, slight puncture of the liver or kidney results in haematoma formation which usually resolves within a few days. Penetration of the gizzard is unlikely in the herbivorous birds because of its thick-walled nature, but in carnivorous birds the gizzard has a much thinner wall and is much more likely to rupture, particularly if the bird has not been starved for 24 hours prior to laparoscopy. However, before starving the bird, the clinician should take account of the bird's nutritional state because of the danger of hypoglycaemia. If the gizzard is punctured this will necessitate a laporotomy and suturing the organ, together with appropriate antibiotic cover. In the case of all sites of entry there is a slight risk of subcutaneous emphysema through air leaking from the air sac system but this usually resolves spontaneously.

Apart from these hazards the technique is not as easy as it might at first appear and much practice is required to develop the necessary skill, particularly in the smaller birds. The practitioner would therefore be wise to learn this art on several freshly-killed cadavers before proceeding to the live bird. One of the first difficulties of an unskilled operator is failure to obtain a clear sighting of the internal organs when looking down the telescope. One may see nothing more than an opaque pale-pink haze. This usually means that the tip of the endoscope is lying against one of the viscera or its view is obscured by air sac or peritoneal membrane or it has not properly penetrated the abdominal muscles. Very slight and slow retraction of the endoscope and cannula or slight withdrawal of the endoscope into the cannula, often results in the view clearing. If nothing happens the instrument should be pulled further back and if there is no improvement then it is likely that the abdominal muscle has not been penetrated. The endoscope should be removed and the trocar reinserted and the direction of the penetration reassessed.

If the internal organs can be dimly seen but they are not clear then the operator is looking through an air sac membrane. Air sacs vary in their clarity and it may be possible for the experienced clinician to identify an ovary or testes without proceeding further. However, to obtain a clearer view, the posterior abdominal membrane will have to be ruptured. It may be possible to do this by simply advancing the endoscope and cannula and at the same time giving a slight twist. However, it might also be necessary to reinsert the trocar.

If the view down the endoscope is obscured by a blood red haze, then a blood vessel has been ruptured or the liver or kidney has been penetrated. It is safer to cease the operation for a short period until the situation can be evaluated. If the endoscope is only partially obscured by blood this can often be wiped free against a suitable internal organ such as the gizzard.

Another problem is excess abdominal fat. This is not uncommonly found in captive, inactive raptors. Also the abdomen may be partly filled with exudate as in the case of an egg peritonitis.

Having penetrated the abdomen and obtained a clear view, the next problem experienced by the unskilled operator is orientation of the various organs in relation to each other. The operator must learn to appreciate that slightly advancing or withdrawing the endoscope makes a relatively rapid change in the magnification of the object being viewed.

Examination of the internal organs

The first organs usually to be seen and which are unlikely to be mistaken by anyone who has carried out a number of avian post mortems are the lungs. The caudal ventral surface of these structures can be examined and the ostia of the secondary bronchi where these enter the caudal thoracic air sac can be seen. Depending on which site of entry is used, the endoscope may have entered the caudal thoracic or the abdominal air sac. It may be necessary to puncture the division between these two air sacs to see other organs clearly. Lying ventral to the lungs (to the left in the recumbent bird) the pulsating heart can easily be recognized. Moving the tip of the endoscope further to the operator's left, the lobes of the liver can be seen as they approach the heart and partially envelope the gizzard. If the endoscope is then carefully moved to find the medial caudal edge of the left lung, the large rounded dark brownish-red colour of the left cranial division of the kidney can be recognized. This lies posterior but very close to the lung. Immediately ventral and slightly anterior to the kidney is situated the pink-coloured adrenal gland. The gonads lie adjacent but caudal to the adrenal gland, so that the kidney, adrenal and gonads form the 3 points of a triangle.

Surgical sexing

In the immature male the testis is a rounded, slightly oval structure very little bigger than the adrenal gland but a little more yellow in colour. In some species the testes may be wholly or partly pigmented dark green or black in colour. In the immature bird it may be possible to see both testes lying one on each side of the dorsal aorta and vena cava. As the testis matures, it increases in size and blood vessels become obvious on the surface. The blood vessels become more tortuous with age. In the active testes during the breeding season the organ may become very large and more difficult to recognize. In the

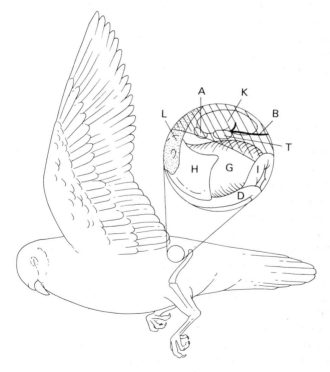

Fig. 2.5. Organs that can be identified by laparoscopy. ▨ indicates the extent of the abdominal air sac. A, adrenal gland; B, main blood vessels; D, duodenum; G, gizzard; H, liver; I, intestine; K, kidney; L, lung; T, testis.

aged testis the gonad is more angular in shape. In the immature female the ovary tends to be 'L' shaped and about the same length as the cranial division of the left kidney. The colour is a buff yellow, the surface is flat and the texture slightly granular in appearance. Sometimes the ovary is pigmented. As the ovary matures follicles become more apparent and these will vary in size. Gradually as the ovary increases in size it begins to obscure the kidney and adrenal gland. In the active ovary during the breeding season some of the individual follicles can become very large, taking up a large part of the abdominal cavity. In the old female bird the ovary has contracted again and whilst follicles can be recognized much of the ovary is occupied by scar tissue.

At the end of laparoscopy the skin and underlying muscle are brought together with a single suture. Some operators consider this unnecessary. Bush (1980) describes the taking of biopsy specimens under direct vision, using a secondary cannula with biopsy forceps or using a biopsy needle, to aid in the early diagnosis of tuberculosis of the liver. Samples can also be taken from other organs for culture and histopathology. Fluids can be aspirated from an air sac under direct vision or small quantities (3 ml in a large bird) of fluid can be instilled into the air sacs to obtain sample washings.

Other uses for the endoscope

The instrument can also be used to examine the posterior part of the nasal cavity through the choanal opening. The trachea, the syrinx and bronchi may also be inspected. Before the latter is examined the posterior air sacs are cannulated to allow unobstructed respiration to proceed. The ease with which all these cavities can be viewed will obviously depend on the size of the bird. It is also possible to visualize the oesophagus, crop and proventriculus of a bird as small in weight as 40 g.

Laparoscopic photography

Special cameras can be used for clinical documentation of the organs viewed through the endoscope. Adaptors can also be obtained so that the telescope eyepiece can be coupled to the standard lens of any single lens reflex camera. The best results are obtained if a xenon flash tube is incorporated in the light source but this increases the initial cost of the equipment. For photography it is better to use a 5 mm-diameter endoscope which transmits more light than the smaller diameter instruments—less exposure of the film being necessary. Nevertheless, it is possible to obtain reasonably good results with a 2.7 mm-diameter endoscope, using Kodachrome 64 (ISO.64) film, with exposures of the order of .25–.50 second. One needs a steady hand, good anaesthesia and an assistant to operate the shutter of the camera with a cable release. The camera lens is focused at infinity and set to maximum aperture before coupling to the endoscope. If the camera has interchangeable viewing screens a clear screen is best.

Radiography

This is a useful aid to diagnosis particularly in the case of abnormalities of the skeleton, but also in disease of other organ systems.

Restraint of the avian patient

To obtain good results, radiography is best carried out under general anaesthesia or at least deep sedation. This enables the radiographer to position the bird carefully with correct centering and collimation of the X-ray beam. It is possible to take quick radiographs of the extremities of a hand-held bird, but apart from the risks to the handler, it is almost impossible to adequately and gently restrain a small bird whilst wearing protective lead rubber gloves. Having attained anaesthesia or deep sedation the patient is best maintained in the required position using adhesive plaster or Sellotape placed over the limbs and neck.

Radiographs, to be of maximum diagnostic value, should be obtained only after care has been exercised to obtain a true dorsal/ventral or lateral position of the patient. This is tedious and needs meticulous assessment by the operator to judge by sight and touch that the sternum overlies the vertebrae. If correct positioning is not achieved in the dorsal/ventral position, the two sides of the body cannot be accurately compared. Apparent distortion of various structures and body cavities may be seen which have no clinical significance. The air sacs on one side may look smaller than those on the other side of the body. The shadow of the liver and the position of the gizzard may become distorted. In the true lateral position the two hip joints and the two shoulder joints should overlap. The wings must be held by the tape above the body and the legs must be extended as far back as possible.

When X-raying the wings care should be taken, not only to have both wings in a flat position and as close to the X-ray film as possible, but also to make sure that both wings are extended to the same degree. It is very helpful in making a diagnosis to be able to compare the radiographic image of the two wings. As the shoulder joint extends, slight rotation of the humerus takes place and as the elbow joint extends, the radius slides longitudinally in relation to the ulna. Also an extension of the carpal joint, pronation of the metacarpal region occurs.

Radiographs of the skull should be in true dorso/ventral and lateral positions with the neck fully extended.

X-ray film and exposure factors

Radiographs may be taken on X-ray film held in the cassettes preferably with fast calcium tungstate or rare-earth intensifying screens. Alternatively, non-screen film may be used to obtain greater detail. Using Ilford red seal film with rare-earth screens at a distance of 36 inches, a kilovoltage of 48 and a milliamp/second (m.a.s.) value of 4, is found to be satisfactory for a bird the size of a budgerigar. For somewhat larger birds of about 400 g (e.g. African grey parrot) the kV. should be increased to 58. McMillan (1982a) suggests increasing these kV. values by 10 units, and so halving the m.a.s. value.

When using non-screen film, the focus to subject distance can be reduced to 20 inches. This will reduce the exposure time necessary and in the case of small birds there will be very little loss of image quality due to distortion. Using a kilovoltage of 48 the m.a.s. value should be approximately 50 for a budgerigar. Alternatively if the kV. is increased to 90 the m.a.s. can be reduced to 9. There is some reduction in contrast but for many purposes the radiograph obtained is quite useful.

The radiographer should be aware that there is considerable difference in size in the air sacs between the inspiratory and expiratory phases of respiration. If possible the exposure is best made at the end of the inspiratory pause when the air sacs are at maximum dilation so that optimal use is made of the natural air contrast in the avian body.

No grid is necessary since most avian bodies are less than 10 cm in thickness and the total mass of tissues is less than in mammals of comparable size.

Radiographs of the muscle/skeletal system

Radiography is an aid to avian orthopaedic surgery, and is helpful in assessing the degree of distortion and prognosis in metabolic bone disease. Osteoporosis is most often but not only seen in raptors. It occurs in fledglings which have not received a balanced calcium phosphorous intake which should be about 1.5:1.0. This results in folding distortion of the thin and weak cortex of the long bones. Gross distortion of the bones in the wings and legs takes place which often results in the bird becoming a permanent cripple. The disease is most likely to occur in the case of artificially-reared birds of prey fed entirely on a diet of meat, which contains little if any calcium. It also occurs in wild birds. Other conditions that can be recognized by radiography include, osteomyelitis, neoplasia and arthritis. This is sometimes seen in pigeons, in the carpal and shoulder joints, with *Salmonella* infection. Radiography of all the limb joints in the bird is easy except in the case of the hip joint where the shape of the ilium makes outlining of the joint difficult.

Another condition, often found incidently during radiography is polystotic hyperostosis. This is not uncommon in the budgerigar and is also occasionally seen in other psittacines. It is recognized by the medullary cavities of the long bones—normally filled with air—becoming filled with solid bone. There is also a general overall increase in bone density throughout the skeleton. The disease is believed to be due to excess oestrogen and can be reproduced by a stilboestrol implant (McMillan, 1982b).

When viewing radiographs of the skeleton in the diagnosis of orthopaedic problems, one should try and get as much information as possible about the muscular system. A reduction in size of one of the pectoralis muscles due to muscle atrophy, can often be seen on a radiograph though it may not be so obvious by palpation. It may be possible to detect slight contraction and swelling of the muscle mass of the supracoroideus after rupture of the tendon that passes through the foramen triosseum. In the forelimb, the shadows of the biceps and triceps brachii muscles can be identified. A large part of the latter muscle originates from the surface of the humerus and is liable to sustain trauma in fracture of the adjacent bone. The tensor muscles and tendon of the propatagial membrane are often damaged. This may result from collison with such objects as telephone wires. The flexors and extensors of the carpus and digits should be examined.

Signs of injury to muscles are shown by a subtle increase in density when compared with the other wing. Some idea of how recent an injury to the skeleton is, can be gauged by the condition of the neighbouring muscles. In a very recent injury there is a noticeable increase in size and density of the radiographic shadow. This usually decreases considerably, almost returning to normal during the course of the next few days, providing the fracture is not compound and there is no superimposed infection.

Interpretation of soft tissue radiographs

Since the radiograph is a two dimensional shadow of a three dimensional structure, it is essential to take both dorsal/ventral and lateral views when X-raying the internal organs. Whereas the air sacs provide some natural contrast, it is still essential to make a correct exposure if one is to gain the maximum information from the radiograph. Also, if possible the exposure should be made at maximum inspiration.

One of the most obvious features to be seen when first looking at an avian dorsal/ventral (d/v) radiograph is the 'waist' between the shadow of the heart and that of the liver. If the two shadows become indistinct and merge into one uniform outline, this usually indicates hepatomegaly. Alternatively, a reduction in size due to atrophy of the liver may be recognized. If the liver is enlarged, in the d/v view the gizzard is often seen to be displaced well to the left-hand side and in the lateral view to be displaced caudally and slightly dorsally. The gizzard is easily recognizable in granivorous birds because of the retained grit and normally occupies a position just to the left of the mid-line. If a bird has been given only soluble oyster shell grit, then the gizzard may not be identified by this method. Also a bird may have been deprived of grit. Space-occupying lesions may be responsible for displacing the normal position of the gizzard shadow. Enlargement of the gonads, which occupy a position ventral to the anterior of the kidney and the syncrosacrum, may, if greatly enlarged, displace the gizzard. This is normal in the breeding season. In lesions of the oviduct, such as a gross salpingitis and impaction with inspissated

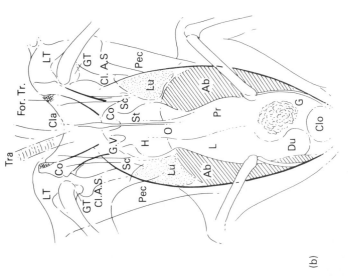

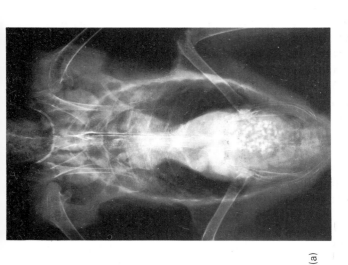

Fig. 2.6. (a) Ventro-dorsal radiograph of Festive Amazon Parrot. (b) Ab, abdominal air sac; Cla, clavicle; Clo, cloaca; Cl.A.S., clavicular air sac diverticulum; Co, coracoid; Du, duodenum and supraduodenal loop of intestine; H, heart; For. Tr., foreamen triosseum; G, gizzard; GT, greater tuberosity for the flexor muscles of the shoulder joint; G.V., great blood vessels—the aorta and its branches; L, liver; Lu, lung; LT, lesser tuberosity for the insertion of the supracorocoideus. Immediately behind is the deltoid crest for the insertion of the pectoralis; O, oesophagus; Pr, proventriculus; Pec, pectoralis major muscle; Sc, scapula; St, sternum; Tra, trachea.

yolk, the gizzard will be displaced ventrally and either cranially or caudally. The renal shadow occupies a similar position to that of the gonads but only very rarely is enlargement due to a neoplasm, such as an adenocarcinoma, sufficient to displace the gizzard. This is more apparent if the left kidney is affected. Pathological change in the viscera is often accompanied by a slight increase in density of the radiographic shadow. In species of birds such as raptors where the gizzard is not detectable by its retained grit, the gizzard can be made visible only by using barium sulphate contrast media.

Foreign bodies such as fish hooks, lead shot and nails are not uncommonly seen lodged in the oesophagus, the proventriculus or gizzard of water fowl and are sometimes seen in other species. They may occasionally pass farther along the alimentary canal.

In good quality radiographs the two lungs can be identified by their slight honeycomb appearance. This effect is best seen in the lateral view, and at maximum inspiration. The diagnostician should look for any slight localized increases in density or patches where there is loss of the normal reticular pattern. This indicates fluid or gaseous exudate. The air sacs should be carefully examined. The extra thoracic diverticula of the clavicular sacs can be seen in the pectoral muscle mass around the proximal end of the humerus. In fractures of this bone this part of the air sac system may be damaged as is shown by a change in shape or increase in size or density of the X-ray image. When looking at the abdominal air sacs, absence of their outline may be due to a space-occupying lesion, or more likely due to adhesions or gross air sacculitis. Less severe air sacculitis is recognized by a general haziness of part or all of the air sac spaces. In the lateral view striated dense lines on the radiograph represent the end on view of thickened air sacs. An overall homogenous 'ground glass' increase in density, of both thoracic and abdominal cavities accompanied by obvious distension of the caudal abdomen is usually due to peritonitis. These birds are often in respiratory distress, due to malfunction of the air sac system and are bad anaesthetic risks, particularly if placed in dorsal recumbency. Consequently good X-rays of this condition are not easy to obtain. There are a few inter-species peculiarities of which the avian radiologist should be aware. In the Anatidae (ducks and geese) there is a normal balloon-like irregular distension of the syrinx. This increases in size with age. In swans, cranes, spoonbills and birds of paradise, the trachea is elongated into coils which lie between the skin and pectoral muscles or within a tunnel in the sternum (King & McLelland, 1975a). In penguins the trachea is bifurcated for most of its length.

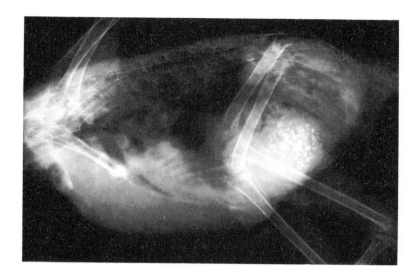

(a)

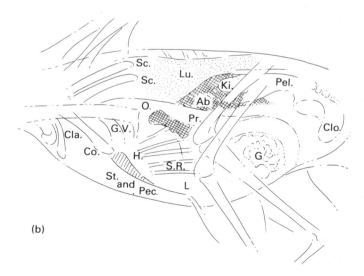

(b)

Fig. 2.7. (a) Lateral radiograph of a Festive Amazon Parrot, (b) Ab, abdominal air sac; Cla, clavicle; Clo, cloaca; Co, coracoid; G, gizzard; GV, great vessels; H, heart; Ki, kidney; Lu, lung; L, liver; O, oesophagus; Pel, pelvis; Pr, proventriculus; Pec, pectoralis muscle; Sc, scapula; St, sternum; SR, sternal ribs.

The use of contrast media

Contrast radiography of the alimentary canal

Barium sulphate suspension can be placed in the crop by an oesophageal tube made from any suitable diameter plastic or rubber tubing fitted to the nozzle of a hypodermic syringe. A rigid metal catheter, smooth at the distal end, can also be utilized for birds such as psittacines which are liable to nip off a softer tube. When using a rigid tube, it should be well lubricated. After extending the bird's head in a vertical direction, allow the tube to slide down under its own weight. The barium sulphate is best diluted with an equal quantity of water and then flushed down with water. A suitable quantity of diluted barium sulphate for a budgerigar is 0.5 ml, followed by another 0.5 ml of water. For a bird the size of an African Grey Parrot 2 ml amounts would be reasonable. Give the suspension slowly to avoid reflux up into the pharynx. The time taken for the contrast media to reach the various parts of the alimentary canal will depend on any drugs used for premedication and anaesthesia and also on any pathological condition that may be present. On average the barium will have reached the proventriculus and gizzard within 5 minutes and be in the small intestine within 30 minutes. Contrast media can help to define the position of the alimentary canal relative to the other viscera. It should reach the cloaca in about 3 hours. Barium sulphate suspension or one of the iodine contrast agents such as meglumine iothalamate* 70%w/v or sodium diatrizoate† 45%w/v can be used for an enema to outline the cloaca and rectum. Suitable amounts of the contrast agents for this technique in an Amazon Parrot would be 1.5 ml of diluted barium sulphate followed by 3.5 ml of water. Air may be used as an alternative in the crop. Approximately 3 ml of air are required for this purpose in the budgerigar.

Bronchography

One of the iodinated water-soluble contrast mediums can be used to outline the primary and secondary bronchi in the avian respiratory system. The procedure is carried out in the

* Conray 420
† Hypaque 45%

anaesthetized bird held in the lateral position. It is safer to first catheterize the posterior air sacs by the method described for laporoscopy. In this way an unobstructed airway is maintained to the respiratory system. The contrast agent is then introduced by a fine 16-gauge or 1 mm nylon catheter, similar to those used for intravenous cannulation, into the lower part of the trachea, stopping just cranial to the syrinx. The syrinx and the bifurcation of the trachea into the 2 primary bronchi is situated, in most species of birds, just caudal to a line joining the two shoulder joints. If the cannula is introduced beyond this point there is a possibility that it will enter one or other of the primary bronchi.

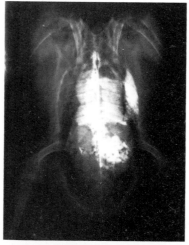

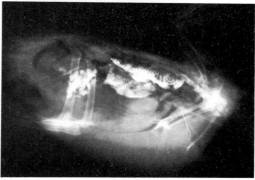

Fig. 2.8. Bronchogram of the lungs of a pigeon (*Columba livia*).

Because of the diamter of the trachea the technique has only been used by the author in birds of above 300 g in body weight. A suitable quantity of contrast agent for a 400 g bird (e.g. Amazon parrot) is 1 ml. If the bird is in lateral recumbency and the contrast agent is introduced slowly, it will tend to enter the lower primary bronchus because of gravitation. Bronchography is carried out on one side at a time.

Urography and angiocardiography

The iodinized water soluble contrast agents mentioned above can be injected intravenously and will outline the heart and kidneys. For a bird the size of an Amazon parrot 1/ml should be given by slow injection and the radiograph for the heart taken immediately the injection is finished. If it is required to outline the kidney the X-ray should be taken after 5 minutes.

Cealiography

McMillan (1982c) describes a method of outlining the viscera in the budgerigar, by injecting 0.2 ml of sodium diatrizoate into the abdomen.

3 / Post-mortem Examination

There is probably no other way in which a clinician's acumen is increased than by post-mortem examination. The post-mortem of patients subsequent to an ante-mortem diagnosis will help increase the practitioner's diagnostic ability and indicate ways in which the diagnostic routine can be improved.

The owner of a single bird, be it a pet cage bird or a falconer's hawk, is often interested in the cause of death and if there was anything he could have done to prevent death.

The client who has a flock of wild fowl or an aviary of birds that are chronically sick is often willing to sacrifice one or a few birds to establish the cause of the problem.

To be of maximum value post-mortem specimens should be as fresh as possible. However, sometimes a client will produce a carcass in which death occurred 24–36 hours previously. In this case the carcass should be thoroughly soaked with cold water and placed in a plastic bag with any excess air expressed. The sealed bag should then be put in a refrigerator so that the body is kept at a temperature just above freezing but not frozen. The feathering helps to retain body heat, so cooling the body as quickly as possible will help to reduce autolytic changes. If the carcass is deep-frozen the fine cellular structures are ruptured by ice crystals. Such tissues are useless for histopathology.

In those specimens that are up to 3 days old and in which no precautions have been taken to prevent autolylis, some useful information may often still be obtained.

A post-mortem should always be carried out in a systematic and routine order so that nothing is overlooked or forgotten. Having a check list to hand is invaluable.

The practitioner should realize that the gross lesions seen during post-mortem can only provide a tentative diagnosis. Further laboratory tests will be needed for confirmation in most cases. Therefore it is wise to have certain equipment ready before starting the autopsy.

Some equipment that may be required during a post-mortem examination together with an indication of the laboratory techniques that can be used.

(1)   A check-list of organs to be examined.

(2)   Scalpel and blades.

(3)   Rat-toothed forceps.

(4)   Sharp-pointed dissecting scissors.

(5)   Spirit lamp or Bunsen burner.

(6)   Bacteriological culture plates, blood agar and MacConkey agar.

(7)   Bacteriological swabs.

(8)   Transport media. All living specimens have a better chance of survival if placed in transport media.

(9)   Screw-top containers with 10% formol saline that should preferably be buffered. When harvesting solid organs specimens should not be more than 0.5 cm thick, otherwise the formaline will not fully penetrate the tissue. At least 10 times the volume of preservative as the specimen is required.

(10)   Screw-top sterile containers to contain tissues for bacteriological culture.

(11)   Slides. These can be used for:

   (a)   bacteriological staining; if the slide is sterilized by heating in the flame, the bacteriological swab will remain uncontaminated after the smear has been made on the sterile slide.

   (b)   slides can be used to make impression smears from liver, spleen and air sacs. Liver smears can be stained with modified Ziehl-Neelsen or Macchiavello's stain for chlamydia inclusion bodies or with haematoxylin and eosin for herpes virus inclusion bodies seen in some species.

   (c)   if the bacteriological swab is rolled along the sterile slide instead of smearing across it, it can be stained with Wright's or Leishman's stain and then used for cytological examination.

(12)   Strong scissors or even bone forceps for large birds.

(13)   Some sterile gauze swabs are sometimes useful if a blood vessel is inadvertently punctured.

(14)   Sterile syringes and needles for the sterile collection of heart, blood and intesinal contents for culture. If the ingesta are too viscid, a little sterile normal saline injected into the lumen of the gut will make them more fluid. To collect sterile samples from the interior of unopened hollow organs, first sterilize the surface by searing with a hot spatula before inserting the needle.

(15)   At least one pair of sterile petri dishes to collect tissues for virus isolation, as suggested by Harrison & Herron (1984).

(16)   Good lighting possibly combined with a magnifying lens is a great help.

(17)   A suitable board and dissecting needles for pinning out small birds.

Always wear gloves and a mask. Apart from the risks of chlamydia infection, which is not confined to parrots and is not uncommon in ducks and pigeons, there are many other avian zoonoses.

External examination

Before starting the post-mortem it may be helpful to X-ray the carcass, if for instance, it was suspected the bird was shot or suffering from metabolic bone disease or was involved in some sort of accident.

Prior to opening the body a thorough examination should be carried out looking for any of the external signs described in Chapter 1. External parasites are often a lot more obvious on the dead body as they move away from the cooling surface of the skin. The specimen should next be saturated with a quaternary ammonium antiseptic. This reduces the amount of airborne feather debris. Feather dust can carry chlamydia and other organisms and also contaminates the viscera when the carcass is opened.

The body is next pinned out on a board. Plucking the whole body is unnecessary. The removal of feathers along the mid-line in densely feathered species, such as ducks and gannets, does help to make it easier to incise the skin cleanly without damaging the underlying viscera.

Opening the body

The initial incision is made through the skin from the cranial end of the sternum to just in front of the vent. The cut is then extended on each side just along the caudal edge of the sternal plate. By blunt dissection the skin is then eased away from the underlying pectoralis muscle and at the same time the condition of the muscle is observed.

The pectoralis muscle

Both sides should be similar and well-rounded. If the two muscles are not symmetrical it may indicate an old injury or an inspissated and contracted abscess. The muscle should be of normal red colour showing no sign of anaemia, hyperaemia or bruising. The latter may be anything from bluish-black to green (within 24 hours) in colour

depending on how long previously the bruise occurred. Discolouration of abdominal muscles also may occur if they have had prolonged
contact after death with the gut or gall bladder (if this was displaced
caudally). Bacterial invasion from the gut into the surrounding tissue
can be relatively rapid in the uncooled carcass.

Incise the pectoralis muscle and look for any evidence of petechial
haemorrhages in the muscle which could indicate Warfarin poisoning
(Reece, 1982) or vitamin K deficiency. Note the observations of
Fiennes (1969) mentioned in the section dealing with disease of
the lower alimentary canal (p. 51).

Exposing the viscera

The skin incisions are now deepened through the muscle and the
lateral incisions are now extended to the level of the costochondral
junctions which are either cut with scissors, or, in small birds,
dislocated by pressure from the handle of a scalpel. Do not cut
through the coracoids or clavicles at this stage, as this may damage the
large blood vessels leaving the heart. The sternum now can be lifted
upwards away from the underlying viscera. As this is done examine
the underside (anatomically the dorsal aspect) of the sternum together
with the general appearance of the organs. If the body cavity is filled
with exudate, take swabs for culture. Decide if the colour of the
tissues looks a normal pink or is hyperaemic indicating a possible
septicaemia. Discolouration, due to hypostatic congestion, on one
side only, would indicate the bird had been left for some time lying on
that side after death.

The carcass may look anaemic. Even if heavy infestation with
blood-sucking parasites had been noticed initially, there may also be
other less obvious contributing factors. The muscle may look dry
indicating dehydration or shrunken indicating cachexia.

Examination of the viscera before removal from the body

The signs of air sacculitis may be seen and will become more evident
as the post-mortem proceeds. During the initial stages of air sacculitis
the crystal-like clarity of these delicate sheets of tissue is lost. They
become increasingly opaque and thickened as exudate begins to
collect between their 2 layers of cells. At first this cloudiness is patchy
but later extends through the whole system of air sacs. Yellow caseous

material becomes more evident. There may be a varying distribution of discreet disc-like plaques which show a necrotic centre. These may indicate *Aspergillus* infection and diagnosis should be confirmed by taking a swab for culture and microscopical examination. An impression smear can also be taken and stained with Gram's stain or lactophenol blue when mycelia and the club-shaped fruiting heads can be seen, particularly at the edge of the specimen. In air sacculitis due to *E. coli*, the thickened parts of air sac and caseation tend to be more generalized and irregular in shape.

Occasionally at this stage of the post-mortem the organs can be seen to be covered with a scintillating sheen of urate crystals indicating visceral gout. The minute black mites of the genus *Sternostoma* may be seen in the air sacs particularly of finches. Occasionally in falcons nematodes of the genus *Serratospiculum* may be seen (Cooper, 1978).

The liver

If the liver is ruptured and is accompanied by a large blood clot this could be due to a blow over the sternum. In this case there will usually be signs of bruising of the overlying muscle and skin. The liver may be bile-stained (in those species which have a gall bladder—it is absent in many pigeons and parrots) due to bile diffusion from the gall bladder through the dead tissue of the bladder wall—a process which takes place within a few hours of death. The liver may be enlarged, and in fatty livers rupture will occur easily without any external trauma. Enlargement of the liver is indicated by loss of the normal sharp edges which become rounded. If this is accompanied by faint areas of necrosis which are seen at the same time as a fibrinous or serous pericarditis and air sacculitis, death may have been due to chlamydia (psittacosis) infection. An impression smear of the liver stained with either a modified Ziehl-Neelsen stain (see Chapter 2, p. 25) or Macchiavello's stain, may show the pink intracytoplasmic inclusion bodies. Also in chlamydia infection the spleen will be enlarged or distorted in shape or possibly ruptured.

Pacheco's parrot disease may cause liver lesions that mimic chlamydia infection. These lesions tend to be more saucer-shaped and cause a faint yellow discolouration which stands out against the mahogany-coloured liver. Other herpes viruses affect other groups of birds and can cause necrotic foci in the liver. Principal amongst these is the disease in falcons, storks and cranes. Pigeons can also be affected by a herpes virus but this attacks mainly the young birds. In owls, herpes virus liver lesions look more like avian tuberculosis, with small white or yellowish pustules up to the size of a pea and possibly not raised above the surrounding surface. Some of the other organs may be covered by these lesions. Avian tuberculosis should not be confused with the pin head necrotic foci of *Salmonella*, *E. coli* or *Pasteurella*. A swab stained with Ziehl-Neelsen and Gram's stain may identify the organism. Fiennes (1969) describes the liver as being a rich golden colour and somewhat fatty in the case of septicaemic *Salmonella* infection.

In turkeys and game birds the black, circular lesions of blackhead due to histomoniasis infection may be found. If the liver is mottled with irregular, lighter-coloured areas this may be neoplasia.

If at this initial examination of the viscera there are signs of a septicaemia, a sterile specimen of heart blood should be taken. The surface of the organ is first sterilized by searing with the blade of a hot spatula. A sterile needle attached to a syringe is then inserted into the heart for the withdrawal of blood.

If the bird has not long been dead it may be possible to make a smear and look for blood parasites. The blood obtained should also be cultured and stained with Gram's stain.

Removal and examination of the alimentary canal and spleen

This should be carried out by cutting the lower oesophagus or proventriculus and incising the skin around the vent. The cloaca and the attached bursa of Fabricius should be removed intact and care should be taken not to contaminate the rest of the carcass. The spleen should be attached to the underside of the caudal end of the proventriculus (anatomically the dorsal side).

The spleen

The spleen is globular in most species but may be triangular in ducks and geese and is usually about one quarter to one third the size of the heart. Never ignore an enlarged or angular-shaped spleen or one that may have ruptured. It may indicate chlamydia infection. The spleen may be slightly enlarged and hyperaemic due to a septicaemic infection or, as in the case of the liver, mottled with the foci of a neoplasia. The signs of tuberculosis, *Pasteurella, E. coli* septicaemia and aspergillosis are similar to those seen on the liver.

The lower alimentary canal

Before dissecting out the gut, examine the pancreas which can usually be seen before the alimentary canal is removed from the abdomen. The pancreas should be examined for evidence of atrophy or neoplasia, neither of which is common in birds.

The accompanying duodenum may look congested or distended. Take a sterile sample of the contents, in the same way as harvesting a sterile sample of heart blood.

If the ingesta are too viscid, dilute by injecting a little sterile saline. Examine the sample for *Coccidia,* by Gram's stain and culture. The Gram's stain will enable assessment of the relative numbers of Gram-positive and Gram-negative organisms. The latter should not be predominant in most healthy birds. Look for signs of intestinal haemorrhage, which could be generalized or patchy throughout the intestine. If this is accompanied by pathological signs in other parts of the body it may be an indication of *Newcastle disease.* However, the pathological signs of *Newcastle disease* vary greatly amongst different species and lesions may not be present in any of the viscera. Always look at the pattern of pathological change in the intestine together with other changes in the rest of the viscera. A single intestinal haemorrhage may not be due to a bacterial enteritis but rather caused by terminal venous congestion brought on by right heart failure as a result of toxaemia.

Fiennes (1969) has pointed out that sporadic haemorrhage occurring anywhere in the body, both internally and externally and unassociated with any other signs may be due to vitamin K deficiency. Vitamin K is partially synthesized by normal gut flora. This may have been disrupted by disease of the bowels or indiscriminate use of antibiotics. Haemorrhage may be due to Warfarin poisoning as mentioned previously when discussing examination of the pectoralis muscle.

Examine the caeca, these vary considerably in shape and size in different species. They are large and obvious in poultry, in passerines they are small and in pigeons and parrots they are rudimentary. They have lobate ends in the barn owl. In turkeys, chickens and game birds the lesions of blackhead may be seen. The caeca are swollen, the mucosa extensively ulcerated and the lumen contains a lot of necrotic material. In *Salmonella* infection, the caecal wall may have a white, glistening appearance.

After an external examination of the bowel the whole alimentary canal should be opened to expose the lumen. The interior may be filled only with a green fluid without any ingesta indicating anorexia. The lower intestine may contain grit from the gizzard indicating increased peristalsis. The mucosa of the bowel may be congested and swollen or flaccid and dilated. If the lumen is filled with catarrhal exudate this could be caused by a parasitic infection. The contents of the bowel and scrapings of the mucosa should be examined for *Coccidia* or *Capillaria* (up to one centimetre long) or helminth eggs. The gut may contain ascarid worms which may be so numerous as to cause impaction and rupture of the bowel.

In the case of *Salmonella* infection the mucosa may show signs of desquamation or show small nodules of necrosis.

Foreign bodies such as fish hooks and small nails are sometimes found in the lumen of the gut and occasionally penetrate the bowel wall.

The proventriculus and ventriculus (or gizzard) should be examined for evidence of the cheesy exudate of *Trichomoniasis* infection which is more commonly found higher up in the alimentary canal.

Signs of *Aspergillus* infection are occasionally found in the lumen of the bowel.

Striations seen in the muscle of the wall of the gizzard may be due to vitamin E deficiency.

Lastly the cloaca together with the bursa of Fabricius should be examined. The latter should be small and involuted in the adult bird. The cloaca may be impacted with urate crystals forming a crumbling calculus or it may be filled with blood clot as the result of damage during artificial insemination. The mucosa of the cloaca can show signs of inflammation or neoplastic change.

Examination of the heart and associated major blood vessels

The exterior of the heart together with the pericardium will already have received some attention when the carcass was first opened but must now be examined in greater detail. The pericardial sac should be examined for any increase in fluid content, the amount of which is normally imperceptible. If the pericardium is unusually opaque this may be caused by infiltration with urate crystals. Examine the myocardium, endocardium and coronary blood vessels for any sign of haemorrhages.

Occasionally the right atrium may be found to be ruptured as a consequence of massive dilation during circulatory failure brought on by an overwhelming disease.

The major blood vessels leaving the heart should be examined. At the same time look for any signs of air sacculitis in the cervicle and interclavicular air sacs. If this is present, it may be productive to cut through the head of the humerus and take a swab from the medullary cavity since this is connected to the anterior air sacs.

When examining the brachiocephalic trunk and the carotid arteries leading away from it, the crop must not be damaged. The interior of the major blood vessels, as well as those of the abdominal aorta and renal arteries, may show atheromatous plaques and these may be so extensive as to apparently occlude the lumen of the vessel.

These lesions are not uncommon in anseriformes, falciformes and ostriches. They are occasionally found in many other species such as psittacines. Young turkeys commonly suffer from dissecting aneurysms of the arteries, which can lead to sudden death.

After the crop has been carefully dissected to one side, in order to examine the carotid arteries, the thyroids and parathyroids should be examined (Fig. 3.1).

Examination of the thyroid and parathyroid glands

Enlargement of the thyroid is not uncommon in budgerigars and is usually caused by iodine deficiency. Neoplasia of the thyroid is not common in birds but a number of clinicians have reported seeing occasional cases when the signs exhibited prior to death are similar to those of thyroid dysplasia. Secondary hyperparathyroidism occurs in birds that have been fed almost entirely on seed that contains very little calcium but excess phosphorous (p. 37). If these birds have been deprived of soluble grit metabolic osteodystrophy may follow.

Examination of the crop

Normally the crop wall is quite thin—in small birds as delicate as tissue paper. However, where there is infection, as with *Candida* or

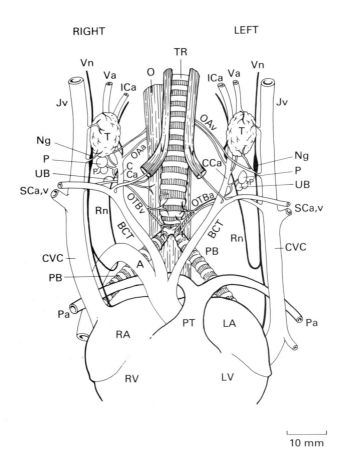

Fig. 3.1. Ventral view of the blood vessels, nerves and glands at the thoracic inlet of the domestic fowl. The carotid bodies are on the medial surfaces of the parathyroid glands. A, aorta; BCT, brachiocephalic trunk; CCa, common carotid artery; CVC, cranial vena cava; ICa, internal carotid artery; Jv, jugular vein; LA, left atrium; LV, left ventricle; Ng, nodose (distal vagal) ganglion; O, oesophagus; OAa, ascending oesophageal artery; OAv, ascending oesophageal vein; OTBa, oesophagotracheobronchial artery; OTBv, oesophagotracheobronchial vein; P, cranial parathryoid gland; P′, caudal parathyroid gland; Pa, pulmonary artery; PB, primary bronchus; PT, pulmonary trunk; RA, right atrium; Rn, recurrent nerve; RV, right ventricle; SCa, subclavian artery; SCv, subclavian vein; T, thyroid gland; TR, trachea; UB, ultimobranchial body or gland; Va, vertebral artery; Vn, vagus nerve. After Abdel-Magied & King (1978), with kind permission of the editor of the *Journal of Anatomy.*

trichomoniasis, the mucosa of the crop can become hypertrophied and noticeably thick. If the white, caseous exudate of *Candida* is scraped from the mucosa, the surface will look rather like velvet.

Physiological regurgitation of seed is normal in the budgerigar when feeding nestlings but there is no accompanying hypertrophy of the crop (Baker, J.R., 1984, personal communication). Occasionally a crop will become impacted, a condition affecting all species. The trapped food will ferment with superimposed bacterial infection and inflammation of the crop. The layman's term of 'sour crop' can cover any of the above conditions. Brooks (1982) reports necrosis of the crop wall in a sparrow-hawk leading to a fistula probably caused by a penetrating spicule of bone.

The oesophagus and oropharynx

The whole of the oesophagus should be opened by making a parallel cut with scissors along each side. If a pair of strong scissors or a pair of bone forceps (in large birds) are inserted with one blade in the mouth, the quadrate bone can be cut and the lower jaw disarticulated. The whole of the upper alimentary tract can now be examined. A caseous exudate could indicate trichomaniasis, *Candida* or there may be signs of *Aspergillus*. The signs of all these infections can be confused and diagnosis should be confirmed by laboratory examination. *Trichomonads* are sometimes difficult to find under the microscope. However, if the exudate is incubated overnight in a trichomanad culture medium*, there is no difficulty (Wallis, A.S., 1984; personal communication).

The clinician should be aware that signs of *Trichomoniasis* may be superimposed on an underlying chlamydia infection (de Gruchy, 1983).

Excessive mucus in this region may be indicative of *Capillaria* infection and the worms are sometimes easily seen in the mucus by naked eye although microscopical examination may be necessary.

Abscesses in the mouth of birds, particularly parrots, are not uncommon and may be due to an underlying vitamin A deficiency. However, the small white specks sometimes seen on the roof of the mouth in pigeons (Wallis, A.S., 1984; personal communication) are not considered to be of any clinical significance.

* Oxoid Ltd., Wade Rd., Basingstoke, Hampshire.

Haemorrhage into the choanal space or into the oral cavity may be noticed when the mouth is first opened. This may be as a result of trauma. Both wild and pet birds will fly into window panes. Sparrow-hawks in their enthusiastic pursuit of prey may collide with a solid object.

The respiratory system

The palatine choanal opening

Mites may sometimes be found inhabiting this area. Look for any sign of infection in this region. The upper beak should be cut across just in front of the cere and the sinuses examined. They may contain catarrhal or caseous exudate or there may be a blood clot.

The glottis

There may be signs of inflammatory change along the edges. Open the trachea by making two parallel cuts. The mucosa may be congested or there may be signs of fungal infection. In those birds that feed on invertebrates, and this includes a wide range of species, the nematode *Syngamus* trachea is commonly found particularly in young birds. Occasionally a foreign body is found such as a seed obstructing the trachea. Caseous plaques are not uncommon in the region of the syrinx and may partially occlude the airway.

The lungs

The air sac system has already received attention when first opening the carcass. The lungs should be examined in situ and then carefully eased away from the adjoining ribs using the handle of a scalpel. Look for any evidence of abscessation or haemorrhage. If this is present examine the adjacent rib. There may be signs of a recent or old fracture.

Haemorrhage into the lung substance may be agonal (unorganized clot) and occur as the result of right heart failure. It may also be the result of inflammatory change. If the lung looks solid, try and float a piece in water. If there is pneumonic change the piece of lung will sink.

The gonads, the adrenals and kidneys

First look at these organs in situ. It may then be possible to strip them out in one piece from the 'bed' beneath the syncrosacrum. This is attempted by gripping the fascia just cranial to this group of organs, peeling back gently and easing the organs out with closed scissors.

Both ovaries and testes vary considerably in size according to the maturity of the bird and the breeding season. In both cases there may be total or partial pigmentation of the gonads—which is normal. In the ovary affected with *Salmonella pullorum* disease the follicles instead of being globular may become misshaped and angular. The disease has been diagnosed in many species. Both male and female gonads can undergo neoplastic change. If there are cysts present in the ovary, examine the bones (ribs, vertebrae, sternum, humerus and skull) to see if there is any distortion or increase in solidity. The condition of polyostotic hyperostosis is not uncommon in budgerigars and may occasionally be seen in other birds. It is most often first noticed during radiography.

The adrenal gland closely associated with the cranial end of the gonad is normally a pale-pink colour but it may become hyperaemic during the course of an infection or it may look almost white in colour. The kidney may be hyperaemic together with the rest of the viscera in septicaemic conditions. Alternatively it may be grey in colour, due to cloudy swelling. The kidneys may show any of the signs seen in the liver due to infectious disease mentioned above. The kidney may be pale in colour and tubules may be prominent when impacted with urate crystals. This could be an indication of salt poisoning. Occasionally neoplasms are seen in the avian kidney.

The nervous system

The peripheral nerves

After the kidney examine the nerves of the sciatic plexus where these leave the spinal cord and emerge beneath the syncrosacrum. These nerves together with those of the axillae and the intercostal nerves should be examined for signs of irregular thickening typical of Marek's disease, seen in poultry and ocasionally in falcons, owls and pigeons. Thickening of the nerves may also occur in riboflavin deficiency.

The brain

During removal of the skin covering the head, evidence of subcutaneous haemorrhage may be seen. This is only significant if there has been a lot of bleeding.

Next find the foramen magnum and in small birds insert the blade of a scalpel, in larger birds a pair of strong scissors or bone forceps will be needed. Cut around the cranium on each side and raise the calvarium to expose the brain.

Signs of haemorrhage within the substance of the bone, sometimes quite extensive, are of no significance and are caused by blood extravasated from blood vessels very soon after death. However, an organized blood clot either over or under the meninges or in the substance of the brain is important. This is so, even if the blood is not clotted and may be evidence of concussion, particularly if there is also a matching bruising of the skin, or haemorrhage into the nasal cavities.

The skeleton

Before finishing the post-mortem examine those parts of the skeleton that were not examined when looking for Marek's disease. Open and look particularly at the joints. Greenish discolouration in the muscles around the joints is evidence of bruising. Signs of a septic arthritis of the joints with discharge of exudate may be signs of *Salmonella* infection in pigeons and poultry. The articular cartilage may also show petechia.

Urate crystals may be seen in the joints of those birds affected with visceral gout as well as subcutaneous tophi. For the muroxide test to confirm the presence of urate crystals see Chapter 1, pp. 17–8.

Cut off the head of the femur and sample the medullary cavity for blood-born bacteria and examine the blood corpuscles for signs of any cellular disorder.

4 / Medication and Administration of Drugs

A problem for the busy practitioner in his consulting room is being presented with an obviously sick bird brought in by an anxious and sometimes demanding owner. He is required to reach an instant diagnosis and to initiate appropriate and immediate treatment. Yielding to these pressures, it is all too common amongst practitioners, to assume that the bird is suffering from a bacterial infection and to dispense a soluble antibiotic. This is usually one of the tetracyclines and the owner is told to put some of this in the drinking water each day.

This routine is not only ineffective, it may in fact decrease the chances of the bird's recovery by disturbing the normal bacterial flora of the alimentary canal. In addition it increases the chances of the emergence of antibiotic resistant strains of bacteria and some of these organisms are pathogenic for man.

If the practitioner cannot persuade the client to let him hospitalize the bird so that a more accurate diagnosis can be made, it would be more logical to assume the sick bird is vitamin deficient. The metabolic turnover of the B vitamins is rapid, many birds in captivity are maintained on a restricted diet and some are chronically short of vitamin A. These vitamins can be given safely in the drinking water or by injection and will give the practitioner a little more time in which to make a more considered diagnosis aided by taking samples for laboratory investigation.

Assessing the weight of a bird

To achieve adequate and safe medication an accurate estimate of the bird's weight must be obtained. For small- and medium- sized birds up to 1 kg in weight, a Persolo spring balance, as used by bird ringers and distributed by the British Trust for Ornithology can be used. The bird is placed in a cloth or plastic bag suspended from the balance. If this is not available a mail or letter balance can be used for birds weighing from 30 to 500 g. This is not quite so accurate but will give a reading within a few grams of the true weight. This balance is not accurate enough for birds below 30 g. Larger birds, particularly falcons and some parrots, will sit on a perch attached to the weighing pan of a more robust balance. Falconers often weigh their birds regularly to maintain them in flying condition and may be able to tell the weight of the bird. Ducks, geese and similar birds may be put in a sack, with the head out and the sack tied around the bird's neck.

If for some reason it is not practical to weigh the bird then reference may be made to a table of bird weights. Such a table is included in Appendix 1.

However, the clinician should be aware that weights in normal birds can vary at least 25% on either side of the mean weight for the species. In sick or starved birds the deviation from the average weight could be greater.

Calculating the dose of drugs

Few medicines are marketed specifically for use in birds. Doses are therefore based on clinical reports or have to be extrapolated from the doses advised by the manufacturer for use in dogs and cats. However, birds have a higher metabolic rate than mammals and the rate increases as the size of the creature decreases. There are also differences in metabolic rate between passerine and non-passerine groups of birds. In addition, other factors such as the density of feather covering are involved. In general the higher the metabolic rate the faster are drugs absorbed, metabolized and cleared from the body. Nevertheless, (Bush, Neal & Custer, 1979) have pointed out that there are anomalies to this pattern. The pharmacokinetics of drugs in most species of birds need much more investigation.

If there is not a recommended or proven dose for a particular circumstance then it is best to calculate the dose from the bird's metabolic/effective weight. In general this is derived as an exponential of the body weight raised to the power of 0.75. For example, if the recommended dose of a drug for a cat is 2 mg/kg the dose for a budgerigar weighing 40 g will not be:

$$\frac{40}{1000} \times 2 = 0.08 \text{ mg}$$

But will be:

$$\frac{(40)^{0.75} \times 2}{1000} = \frac{136.79 \times 2}{1000} = 0.273 \text{ mg}$$

which is well over three times as much as the original dose calculated on a weight for weight basis. This of course is the total quantity to be given in 24 hours and will need to be divided into a larger number of fractions to be administered more frequently than is recommended for the cat. Doses given in this book are those used by other clinicians and the author. They are not necessarily based on the metabolic effective weight and may need to be adjusted in the light of future experience.

The administration of drugs

As in the case with mammals medicines may be given to birds by a variety of routes, some of which are more effective and more appropriate to certain disease conditions.

Medication of the drinking water

This is a convenient method when large numbers of birds have to be treated, such as those in a zoological collection or at a quarantine station or in a poultry flock. A number of drugs are formulated for use in poultry by this method. The daily dose has been calculated on the mean water intake of an average bird during 24 hours. At a very rough approximation 150 ml of water is consumed per kilogram of avian body-weight daily. However, there may be at least a 50% increase or decrease on either side of this figure. The water consumption of healthy birds varies considerably depending on bodily condition, ambient temperatures, diet and species. Fruit eaters such as mynah birds and toucans get much of their water from their food. Raptors may not drink very much. Birds whose normal habitat is desert are able to rely almost entirely on metabolic water.

In the diseased bird water consumption will vary even more, not only will this depend on the normal function of the alimentary canal and kidneys but also on the health of the upper respiratory tract. The nasal cavities in the bird are important organs of water conservation. Consequently drugs given by this method must have a wide margin of safety. A bird that is polydipsic could take in much greater amounts of medicament. At best, blood levels of the drug are liable to be irregular. Antibiotics given by this method are at least likely to reach minimal inhibitory concentrations within the lumen of the alimentary canal, providing the bird is drinking some water.

Nevertheless birds are creatures of habit and sensitive to changes in their feeding and watering routine. If the medication colours the water or adds a taste to it the bird is quite likely to refuse to drink and its illness made worse.

There is little doubt that birds have colour vision. The more brightly coloured the plumage of the species the more acute is their perception of colour likely to be.

It was once thought that birds had little sense of taste. Certainly the number of taste buds per unit area is much less in birds than in mammals. Recent work quoted by King & McLelland, (1984c) has shown that, dependent on the species, birds do have a definite sense of taste. Pigeons are apparently more sensitive than the domestic fowl. Bitter-and salt-tasting substances tend to be rejected. Therefore a drug such as Levamisole, with a bitter taste, may not be readily taken by a species with a well-developed sense of taste. Sweet substances such as sugars (but not saccharin) produce variable responses in individual birds. Therefore adding these to medicines to make them more palatable will have varying results.

One advantage to medicating the drinking water of a group of birds with an antibiotic is that it reduces the number of bacterial organisms that may have contaminated the water supply and so limits the spread of infection. Another point in favour of the method is that it is much less stressful for the bird than having to be caught for medication. However, many drugs lose their potency when in solution.

If drugs for water medication are to be dispensed on a regular basis, it is more convenient to have ready-weighed small quantities. These can be added daily to a known quantity of water. Drinking containers for cage birds vary in volume so that it is simpler if the quantities dispensed are sufficient to be added to a common household utensil such as a kitchen measuring jug (500 ml) or a pint milk bottle (568 ml). This is used as a stock solution to keep the drinking container filled. The remainder of the stock solution is discarded. The method is wasteful but the quantities of drug dispensed are small and it is simple for the client. Alternatively, smaller weighed amounts can be dispensed, for example, sufficient to be dissolved in 50 ml of water and at the same time a 10 ml-syringe dispensed so that the client can accurately measure this volume of water.

Oral medication

The same drugs used for medicating the drinking water can be given orally. Also there are a number of human paediatric preparations suitable for oral administration in birds. Galenicals such as liquid paraffin and formulations containing kaolin and bismuth may be used also.

Although it is possible to administer liquid preparations using a syringe, or a dropper (not glass for parrots), or even to let the fluid drip into the mouth from the end of a cocktail stick, it is not very satisfactory. There is a danger of inhalation of the medication and it can be wasteful and messy. It is more sensible to give the preparation using an oesophageal or gavage tube. For many species a piece of soft plastic (used 'drip' tubing) or rubber tubing attached to a hypodermic syringe works well. The length of the tube should be measured against the bird's neck so that when the neck is extended the tube will reach well down to the level of the crop or the thoracic inlet. The diameter of the tube and capacity of the syringe will depend on the size of the bird. Birds the size of small finches (zebra) to swans can be dosed by this method. In the swan a canine stomach tube and a 60 ml plastic syringe are suitable.

In some birds, particularly the parrots, it is imperative to use either a gag or speculum of some kind or a rigid metal catheter. The author prefers the latter since the procedure can then sometimes be accomplished by one person.

During this procedure the bird may need to be restrained by gently wrapping in a towel. Protective gloves may be necessary but can often be dispensed with once the head is controlled. Whilst holding the beak open, the neck is extended in a vertical direction to straighten out the typical avian s-shape curve of the cervical vertebrae. Having placed the lubricated, rigid tube in the mouth, it is then advanced beyond the glottis and allowed to slide down the oesophagus under its own weight. No stomach tube should ever be forced down. The avian oesophagus is thin and easily ruptured.

Using this method birds can be accurately dosed and fed if nutrients are added to the medication. Experienced nursing staff and intelligent owners can be instructed to dose birds in this way. However, strict hygiene of the tube, syringe and utensils is necessary. Suitable volumes that can be given by this method are given in Table 4.1.

When giving medication orally or in the drinking water it always should be noted that the absorption of drugs from the gut can be adversely affected by parasitism, a diseased mucosa and nutritional deficiencies. The absorption of some antibiotics such as penicillin, ampicillin and lincocin are reduced in the presence of food. Oxytetracycline has a reduced absorption in the presence of calcium

Table 4.1. Suitable volumes (in ml) for oral medication.

Canary	0.25
Budgerigar	0.5 – 1.0
Lovebirds	1.0 – 3.0
Cockatiel	2 – 4.0
Amazon parrot	5 – 10
African grey parrot	5 – 10
Macaw	10 – 15

and so will be affected if a bird is receiving soluble grit in the diet or the antibiotic is given with antacids.

Medicating the food

Seed impregnated with drugs* is available for small pet birds, up to 100 g (cockatiel size) in body weight. Provided the bird will eat it, it is a convenient method of medication. If the practitioner is dealing with a situation where a large number of birds will need medicating on a regular basis, then it may be possible to get a feed manufacturer to incorporate the desired drug in the pelleted feed. Most psittacines, except the macaws, will accept pelleted food providing it is introduced into the diet gradually over 2 – 3 days.

Parrots will sometimes eat powdered tablets or the powder contents of capsules if these are spread on sweet biscuits or on bread with peanut butter or honey. It may be possible to inject some drugs into fruit such as grapes. Toucans swallow grapes whole without crushing them. Seeds can be coated with a powdered drug by moistening the seed or adding a little corn oil. If given too much oil, the bird becomes coated in it. However, since most seed is dehusked before being swallowed this method of giving drugs is unreliable.

For the prophylactic administration of chlortetracycline to psittacines exposed to *Chlamydia* infection, Ashton & Smith (1984) recommend the following mash: two parts maize and two parts rice with three parts of water cooked to a soft, but not mushy consistency. The drug is added at the rate of 5 mg/g of cooked feed. The food is prepared daily and a little brown sugar and seed is added for

*Ornimed: canary seed impregnated with chloramphenicol, sulphonamides, penicillin or vitamin B_{12} (Laboratory for Applied Biology).

palatability. At a rough approximation most birds eat about one quarter of their weight in food daily.

Intramuscular injection

Undoubtedly this is the most accurate and reasonably safe route for parenteral administration of drugs. Either the pectoralis or the iliotibialis lateralis or biceps femoris muscles of the leg can be used. Both sites have advantages and disadvantages. If injection is made into the pectoralis this must be carried out at the caudal end of the muscles. The veins are better developed at the cranial end of the muscle and there is a much greater chance of accidental intravenous injection. Quite severe inflammatory reaction can occur in the muscle after injection (Cooper, 1983). But this is only likely to be of any consequence with repeated injections at exactly the same site. If the injection is made slightly to one side of the carina or keel of the sternum then the needle is unlikely to go beyond the lateral edge of this bone and penetrate the underlying viscera.

Injections into the leg muscles have the same disadvantages regarding bruising. In addition the large ischiadic nerve may be damaged where it courses down the posterior aspect of the femur. Also injections into the legs may pass through the renal portal system before entering the systemic circulation. This is particularly important with drugs that are excreted through the kidney in an unmetabolized state. Some part of the dose may be partly lost before it has a chance to reach therapeutic blood levels (Coles, 1984b).

For the administration of very small volumes to birds a microlitre syringe, which holds 0.1 ml when filled to capacity and which is marked in 0.001 divisions, is very useful. However, these syringes are expensive and need to be maintained with care. A 1 ml tuberculin syringe divided into 0.01 amounts is much less costly. Many drugs in aqueous solution can be diluted in this syringe to measure very small quantities. With those drugs that cannot be diluted, a microlitre syringe is the only answer.

Subcutaneous injection

This method can be used, but only one or two sites are suitable because the avian skin is not very elastic and fluids tend to leak out through the point of needle puncture. If the area covering the pectoralis muscle is used there is little danger of damage to vital structures but the needle must be advanced well under the skin and only a little fluid can be injected at the site. A much better region is the groin. Greater volumes (2 ml into an African grey parrot) can be injected here and, provided the skin is picked up with forceps before making the injection and the needle is not inserted too far, there is little chance of damaging the nerves and blood vessels beneath. Movement of the bird's leg helps disperse the injection. Dispersion can also be aided by adding hyaluronidase* (half an ampoule or 750 I.V.) to the injection. Another useful site is the skin on the dorsal base of the neck. Care must be taken to hold the loose skin of this area away from the underlying vertebrae and muscles and to make the injection in the mid-line.

The administration of volumes of liquid suitable for fluid therapy in birds is quite practical using these sites.

Intravenous injection

This is more easily given into the brachial vein (Fig. 2.1) but the tarsal vein on the medial surface of the leg can be used in some birds as can the right jugular vein. The latter is useful in small birds. Intravenous injection is not always easy not only because of the small diameter of the vein but also because of the fragility of the vein wall. Haematoma formation after intravenous injection is a common occurence. However, intravenous injection is an effective and important method of treatment in an emergency where a bird's life is threatened by disease.

Intraperitoneal injection

This method has been used by some clinicians but is not without the hazard of entering one of the air sacs. A small volume of fluid is probably of no great consequence and in fact the method is suggested by Clubb (1984) as a method of treating disease of the air sacs.

If the injection is only to reach the peritoneal cavity, the skin and underlying muscle must be picked up by forceps to form a 'tent' slightly to the right of the mid-line. The injection is made into this area with the needle directed almost horizontally thus keeping away from the underlying viscera. If a 16×0.5 mm needle

* Hyalase (Fisons).

is used the injection should go into the ventral hepatic peritoneal cavity (see Fig. 6.6 and the accompanying text in Chapter 6). This procedure is carried out most easily in the sedated bird.

Intratracheal injection

This has been used to treat disease of the respiratory system. In small birds this is most easily carried out by using a mammalian intravenous catheter, cut short and attached to the syringe. The drug is then very slowly introduced into the trachea through the glottis, easily seen on the floor of the oral cavity. The bird's neck needs to be held vertically and slightly extended and the tongue needs to be gently restrained on the floor of the mouth. The method is not practical in the unanasthetized parrot. There will be some coughing but this is usually only temporary. Obviously the volume of fluid must be kept to a minimum though up to 1 ml has been given to pigeons and parrots (400 – 500 g) by this method.

Subconjunctival injections

Very small amounts (0.01 – 0.05 ml) of drugs can be placed under the conjunctiva of the upper eyelid. These are usually antibiotics and steroids and can be very effective when a specific diagnosis has been made. Since the technique requires the bird to be absolutely still, general anaesthesia or deep narcosis is advisable. Long-acting preparations are used for this purpose.

Injections into the infraorbital sinus

This technique is described in the chapter on surgery (Fig. 6.2). The method has been used for many years for treating poultry and is quite applicable to many other types of birds.

Topical applications

The local application of ointments and creams can be used but these should only be applied sparingly using a cotton wool bud. If too much is used the plumage becomes damaged. If larger quantities of ointment have to be used then an Elizabethan collar will be necessary to stop the bird becoming grossly contaminated.

Topical applications which are absorbed or dry quickly such as tinctures are more suitable. Dimethyl suboxide* is a useful preparation applied to the legs and feet of birds. It is rapidly absorbed and may be used as a carrier for other drugs.

Ophthalmic preparations

Ophthalmic ointments can be used but have the same disadvantages as other ointments. Ophthalmic drops are much better but their effect is very short and their use needs constant handling of the bird which is a disadvantage. Subconjunctival injection of slowly absorbed drugs is more effective and less stressful for the bird. The instillation of ophthalmic drops into the nasal cavities for the treatment of sinusitis can be used but direct injection into the infra-orbital sinus is more effective.

Inhalation therapy

A major problem in the treatment of disease of the respiratory system is infection of the air sacs. These thin-walled extensions of the lungs hold about 80% of the volumetric capacity of the respiratory system. The walls are no more than two cells thick and have no blood vessels. There is therefore a large 'dead' space within the bird filled with warm, moist air that is not very accessible to the bird's cellular and humoral defence mechanisms. This area is subject to infection particularly by *Aspergillus* fungi and coliform bacteria. The lungs that have a good blood supply are much less liable to be infected unless challenged by massive infection.

Unfortunately air sacculitis can be present for some time and becomes fairly extensive before outward signs are evident.

Inhalation therapy aims to saturate the air in this dead space and reach the internal surface of the air sacs. To be effective the droplet size of the medication must be below 5 μm in diameter otherwise the droplet does not remain suspended in the air stream long enough to reach the target area. Vaporizing the medication does not work because most of the droplets are too big and condense in the upper respiratory tract. To be effective the drug needs to be administered from a nebulizer into a chamber in which the bird is housed during

* Dermavet (Squibb).

Table 4.2. Suitable doses (in mg) for inhalation therapy, to be diluted in 15 ml of saline and administered over a 30 minute period three or four times a day.

Amphotericin[1]	25–100
Tylosin	150
Chloromycetin succinate	200
Spectinomycin	200
Gentamicin	50–200
Dexamethasone	3

[1] Fungizone (Squibb)

therapy. The drug is mixed with a suitable volume of saline, or better, with a vehicle such as tyloxapol* which aids better dispersion of the medicament. Suitable doses are listed in Table 4.2.

The logical use of antibiotics

No antibiotic should be used unless the clinician is reasonably certain that the bird is suffering from a bacterial infection. However, there is sometimes a rapid deterioration in the condition of a young or small bird challenged by an overwhelming infection. In these circumstances the practitioner may decide to start antibiotic therapy before the results of laboratory tests to confirm his diagnosis become available.

Selection of antibiotic

If the antibiotic is required for systemic use it must be of low toxicity. It should penetrate all the bird's tissues easily and the minimal inhibitory concentration of the drug should be as low as possible. A swab should be taken from the choanal space, the orophanrynx or the cloaca, stained by Gram's method and examined under the microscope. This will at least indicate if the organisms present are mainly Gram-positive or Gram-negative and show their relative numbers. This may indicate whether it is safe to use an antibiotic that is principally active against the one or the other group of bacteria. However, in the first instance, until subsequent laboratory tests are completed, a broad-spectrum antibiotic will usually be chosen.

* Alevaire (Winthrop).

Ampicillin, amoxycillin, trimethoprim combined with a sulphona-
mide and the tetracyclines are all reasonable choices. If given by
injection ampicillin, amoxycillin and the trimethoprim combination
are bacteriocidal but the tetracyclines are only bacteriostatic and rely
on the host's immune response to be effective. If the clinician is
reasonably certain that he is dealing with a respiratory infection,
tylosin or erythromycin (both of which are bacteriostatic) combined
with the tetracyclines would be a good initial choice. However, the
results of more extensive laboratory investigation such as antibiotic-
sensitivity testing from swabs taken before and after starting
antibiotic therapy may show that it is necessary to change the
antibiotic being used.

Chloramphenicol is not a good choice with which to start. Apart
from the possibilities of producing resistance strains of *Salmonella*
organisms, which are not uncommon in birds, the drug may depress
the immune response in a debilitated bird.

Bacteriocidal antibiotics are probably better in the first instance.
These drugs work only on bacteria that are dividing. There is a school
of thought that considers intermittent exposure or less frequent
dosage to be a more effective way of using the antibiotic.
Bacteriostatic antibiotics inhibit bacterial multiplication and give
time for the mobilization of the body's defences. However, the
maintenance of a plasma concentration for several days, well-above
the minimum inhibitory concentration, is essential.

The use of broad-spectrum antibiotics inevitably has some adverse
effect on the host's normal bacterial flora, particularly that inhabiting
the gut. Because of this, once the pathogenic organism causing the
illness is identified, together with its sensitivity to antibiotics, it is
wiser to select an antibiotic that has a narrow range of activity.

If the bacterial flora of the gut is disturbed, then the administration
of natural yogurt-containing *Lactobacillus acidopilus* may help to
restore the balance. This can be given by oesophageal tube at the rate
of 2 ml/kg.

In some cases of chronic infection the rate of maturation of the
t-lymphocytes may be depressed and cell-mediated immunity may be
impaired. In these cases it has been demonstrated in birds and
mammals that Levamisole used intermittently, at a lower dose than
the normal anthelmintic dose, may have a beneficial and sometimes
quite marked effect on the progress of the disease.

The use of drugs unregistered for use in a specific species of animal

Under the Medicines Act 1968 a veterinary surgeon is entitled to use any drugs he considers necessary for the treatment of an animal under his care.

Most of the drugs listed in the following tables have not been given a Veterinary Products Licence for use in birds. Many of these products are for medical use in human patients. However, they have all been used either by the author or by other clinicians working with birds.

Table 4.3. Antibiotics for use in birds: the penicillin group.

The antibiotics of this group are safe and bacteriocidal. They are mostly ionized in plasma (pH 7.4) and are not very lipid-soluble and so do not penetrate well across cell membranes. They are therefore not metabolized and are excreted unchanged through the kidney so that if injected in the legs or given orally some may be lost via the renal portal circulation before reaching target areas.

Antibiotic	Formulation	Route	Dosage	Comment
Penicillin G				
'Crystapen' (Glaxovet)	Sodium Benzyl-Penicillin Soluble powder in vials containing 0.5 mega units (300 mg).	i.m. s.c. i.v.	40,000 units (60 mg)/kg, t.i.d.	Active against most Gram-positive organisms. May be toxic for chicks. Procaine compounds are used in poultry but are considered toxic for small birds—but this may have been due to overdosage.
'Ornimed' (L.A.B.)	Canary seed impregnated with penicillin. 3000 I.V./g.	Oral.	1 capful/1.5 g. 30 g daily.	Useful for small, seed-eating birds up to a cockatiel in size.
Ampicillin				
'Penbritin Injection' (Beecham)	A soluble powder in 2 g vials.	i.m. s.c. i.v.	100 mg/kg every 4 hours. 15 – 20 mg/kg for very large birds.	Active against Gram-positive and some Gram-negative bacteria. It is poorly absorbed from the gut and rapidly excreted.
'Penbritin Suspension' (Beecham)	A stable suspension with 150 mg/ml.		100 mg/kg, b.i.d.	
Amfipen L.A. (Mycofarm)	An oily suspension with aluminium stearate containing 100 mg/ml.	i.m.	200 mg/kg daily.	

Product	Formulation	Route	Dose	Notes
'Penbritin Paediatric' Syrup (Beecham)	A suspension containing 125 mg/5 ml packaged in 100 ml bottles.	Oral.	150–200 mg/kg, t.i.d.	
Amoxycillin				
'Clamoxyl i.v. injection' (Beecham)	A sterile, soluble powder for injection 500 mg per vial for reconstitution in 5 ml water for injection.	i.m. s.c. or i.v.	100 mg/kg, t.i.d.	Less ionized and more lipid-soluble than benzyl penicillin. Good absortion from the gut. Widely distributed in the tissues. Active against a wide range of Gram-positive and Gram-negative organisms, particularly *E. coli*.
'Clamoxyl ready-to-use' injection (Beecham)	A suspension containing 150 mg/ml.	i.m.		
'Clamoxyl Palatable Drops' (Beecham)	750 mg of powder for reconstitution in 12 ml water to produce 15 ml of suspension containing 50 mg/ml.	Oral.	50 mg/kg, t.i.d.	
'Clamoxyl Powder' (Beecham)	Packed in 200 g jars containing 20 g drug including a measure. 1 level measure contains 400 mg drug.	Drinking water, food or orally.	150 mg/kg daily.	
Carbenicillin				
'Pyopen' (Beecham)	Vials containing 1 g powder for reconstitution in 2 ml water for injection 500 mg/ml.	i.v. i.m.	100–200 mg/kg, b.i.d. or t.i.d.	Effective against *Pseudomonas* and *Proteus* species and is synergistic with the aminoglycosides.
Ticarcillin				
'Ticar' (Beecham)	1 g vial of powder for solution.	i.v. i.m.	200 mg/kg, b.i.d. or t.i.d.	Non-toxic. More active than Carbenicillin against *Pseudomonas*. Compatible with aminoglycosides.

73

Table 4.3 (contd.)

Antibiotic	Formulation	Route	Dosage	Comment
The Cephalosporins				
Cephalexin 'Ceporex' (Glaxovet Ltd) **'Keflex'** (Eli Lilly)	Paediatric drops 150 mg/ml.	Oral.	35–50 mg/kg, q.i.d.	Active against many Gram-Positive and Gram-negative bacteria. Active against *E. coli* and *Proteus* but not *Pseudomoras*.
Cephalothin 'Keflin' (Eli Lilly)	1 g ampoules for solution and injection.	i.m.	100 mg/kg, q.i.d.	Active against a range of Gram-positive and Gram-negative organisms including *E. coli* and some *Proteus* species. *Pseudomonas* is resistant.
Cefotaxine 'Claforan' (Roussel)	500 mg vials for solution and injection.	i.m.	50–100 mg/kg, t.i.d.	A broad spectrum antibiotic compatible with the aminoglycosides but which may also be nephrotoxic.

Table 4.4. Antibiotics for use in birds: the aminoglycoside antibiotics.

This group of antibiotics have large, charged molecules, consequently they are not absorbed through cell membranes or absorbed from the gut. They are bactericidal and usually compatible with the penicillins. They are often nephrotoxic, an effect potentiated by diuretics such as Frusemide. They have neuromuscular blocking properties often exacerbated by such anaesthetics as Halothane and Methoxyflurane.

Antibiotic	Formulation	Route	Dosage	Comment
Gentamicin				
'Gentovet' (Arnolds)	A sterile, aqueous solution containing 50 mg/ml.	i.m. Intra-tracheal.	4 mg/kg for pheasants. 10 mg/kg for most psittacines. 30 mg/kg for most small birds. All doses are **given t.i.d.**	Active against a wide range of Gram-positive and Gram-negative organisms including *Pseudomonas*, *Proteus* and *E. coli*. *They have a narrow margin of safety.* Useful for treating respiratory infections. Ensure adequate fluid intake.
		Oral, in drinking water.	40 mg/kg, b.i.d. or t.i.d. 1–5 ml/gallon (U.S.A.) 1.5–6 ml/gallon (U.K.)	
'Genticin' (Nicholas)	Eye drops 0.3% w/v. Sterile aqueous solution.	Eye and into nares.	1 – 2 drops into each eye or nares b.i.d. or t.i.d.	Sinusitis and infection of the nasal chambers.
Streptomycin				
'Dimycin' (Glaxovet)	Sterile, stabilized solution containing 333 mg/ml.	i.m.	15 mg/kg, b.i.d. or t.i.d.	Can be used in poultry and large birds. *Must not be used in small birds—too toxic.*
'Streptovex' (Glaxovet)	A brown-coloured solution containing 1 g/20 ml.	Oral.	15 mg/kg, b.i.d. or t.i.d.	Can be used in all sizes of birds. Often combined with kaolin and sulphonamides. Active against a wide range of enteric organisms.

Table 4.4. (contd.)

Antibiotic	Formulation	Route	Dosage	Comment
Neomycin				
'Neobiotic P Aquadrops' (Upjohn)	A solution containing Neomycin sulphate 50 mg Ph. EUR Methscopolamine bromide (Pamine) 0.12mg.	Oral.	12.5 mg/kg; 0.25 ml/kg	Useful for infections of the gut. Do not overdose because of the anticholinergic agent contained in the formulation.
		Drinking water.	4 drops/150 ml	
Kanamycin				
'Kantrex Paediatric Injection' (Bristol-Meyers)	Injectable sterile aqueous solution containing 75 mg/2 ml.	i.m.	10–20 mg/kg, b.i.d.	A broad spectrum antibiotic similar to Gentamicin. Toxic if the bird is overdosed.
		Drinking water.	1.5–6 ml/gallon (imperial) 1–5 ml/gallon (U.S.A.)	
Tobramycin				
'Nebcin' (Eli Lilly)	Injectable solution containing 20 mg in 2 ml.	i.m.	The same doses as for Gentamicin	Similar to Gentamicin and useful when organisms are resistant to Gentamicin.
Spectinomycin				
'Spectam Injectable' (Ceva)	A sterile solution for injection containing 100 mg/ml.	i.m. s.c. Intra-sinally.	10–45 mg/kg poultry daily; 120 mg/kg small birds	A wide range of activity similar to Gentamicin. Very effective against *Salmonellae* and *Mycoplasma*.
		Drinking water; food.	100 – 200 mg/150 ml or 100 – 200 mg/kg body weight daily	Not absorbed from the gut. Useful for 'sour crop' and diarrhoea. Add one-quarter teaspoonful of honey to increase palatability.
'Spectam Soluble' (Ceva)	A soluble powder containing 100 g/sachet.	Drinking water.	100 g/20 gallons or 90 litres	Only suitable for treatment of large numbers of birds.

Table 4.5. Antibiotics for use in birds: the tetracyclines.

These antibiotics are broad spectrum and not very selective in their range of activity. They are equally effective against Gram-Positive and Gram-negative bacteria, *Mycoplasma*, *Coccidia*, some *Rickettsia* and some viruses. Prolonged use may lead to suppression of the host's normal bacterial flora. They are not well absorbed from the gut in the presence of food or calcium ions. The tetracyclines are relatively non-toxic. These antibiotics are only bacteriostatic and therefore it is important to administer frequently and maintain a level above their minimal inhibitory concentration in the plasma.

Antibiotic	Formulation	Route	Dosage	Comment
Oxytetracycline				
'Oxytetracycline injection' (Glaxovet)	An aqueous solution for injection containing 50 mg/ml.		Birds over 700 g in body weight 20 mg/kg, b.i.d. Birds below 400 g in body weight 80 mg/kg t.i.d.	
'Engemycin 5%' (Mycofarm)	An aqueous solution in polyvinyl/ pyrolidone 50 mg/ml.	i.m. s.c. i.v.		
'Panmycin Aquadrops' (Upjohn)	An aqueous suspension containing 100 mg/ml.	Oral.	Birds over 700 g in body weight 20 mg/kg t.i.d. or q.i.d. Birds below 200 g in body weight 60 mg/kg t.i.d. or q.i.d.	
'Terramycin Soluble Powder' (Pfizer)	A soluble powder containing 55 g/kg. A level measure holding 200 mg is supplied with the pack.	Drinking water and food.	2.5 – 7.5 mg/30 ml 50 – 150 mg/600 ml (pint) 1 mg/oz (30g) of food.	Palatability may be increased by adding honey to the water. Rapidly looses its potency in solution. Therefore must be changed at least every 24 hours Use this as the only source of drinking water.

Table 4.5 (contd.)

Antibiotic	Formulation	Route	Dosage	Comment
'Terramycin Poultry Formula' (Pfizer)	A soluble powder containing 132 g/kg.	Food.	See maker's instructions.	
Chlortetracycline				
'Aureomycin Soluble Powder' (Cyanamide)	A green-tinted soluble powder containing 55 g per kg.	Drinking water, food.	As for Terramycin Soluble Powder 5 mg/g of cooked food daily.	Mix in a mash containing 2 parts of maize, 2 parts of rice, 3 parts of water. Cook to a soft consistency but not mushy. Add brown sugar or honey plus a little added seed to increase palatability. (Ashton, 1984)
'Aureomycin Soluble Oblets' (Cyanamide)	Soluble tablets containing 500 mg.	Feed.	150 mg/kg body weight daily.	
'Ornimed' (L.A.B.)	Impregnated canary seed containing 0.5 mg/1 g of chlortetracycline.	Food.	One capful or 1.5 g daily/30 g bird.	Suitable for small birds up to a cockatiel in size. If given to lovebirds make sure they eat some green food. Do not give normal seen until medicated seed has been eaten but do not leave without seed for more than 10 hours.
Doxycycline				
'Vibramycin' (Pfizer)	Syrup containing 50 mg/5 ml. Capsule containing 100 mg.	Oral.	18–26 mg/kg.	Causes less upset to the normal bacteria of the gut than Chlortetracycline. The drug of choice for treating *Chlamydia* infection.

These antibiotics are mainly active against Gram-positive bacteria and mycoplasma. They are bacteriostatic and therefore not compatible with the penicillins or the aminoglycosides. They are compatible with the tetracyclines. They are relatively non-toxic.

Antibiotic	Formulation	Route	Dosage	Comment
Erythromycin				
'Erythrocin Injectable' (Ceva)	A sterile water miscible solution containing 200 mg/ml.	i.m. s.c.	10 – 25 mg/kg once daily.	Can cause a severe reaction when injected i.m. Useful for the treatment of chronic respiratory infection, air sacculitis, sinusitis and some enteric infections including *Campylobacter*.
'Erythrocin i.v.' (Ceva)	A sterile powder for reconstitution 1 g vial add 20 ml water to produce 5%w/v/50 mg/ml.	Inhalation therapy by nebulization.	1 ml of reconstituted injection in 10 ml normal saline 15 minute treatment t.i.d. or q.i.d.	
'Erythrocin Suspension' (Abbot)	Oral suspension containing 20 mg/ml.	Oral.	Psittacines 40 – 80 mg/kg b.i.d.	
'Erythrocin Soluble' (Ceva)	A soluble powder with erythromycin activity 11.56 g/70 g sachets.	Drinking water.	1 sachet/45 litres/10 gallons.	Only suitable for large flocks of birds.
'Mycosan-T' (Chevita) Univet	A soluble powder containing Erythromycin vitamins, trace elements and arsanilate. Sachets of 7.5 g.	Drinking water.	One sachet in 3 litres of drinking water.	Has been formulated for racing pigeons but has been used in parrots and on raptors.
Tylosin				
'Tylan 50 Injectable' (Elanco)	A sterile 50% injectable solution in propylene glycol containing 50 mg/ml.	i.m.	10–30 mg/kg t.i.d. or q.i.d.	Highly lipid-soluble and well distributed in the tissues. A safe antibiotic with a narrow range of activity against Gram-negative bacteria, *Mycoplasma*, *Pasteurella* and *Chlamydia*. Useful for upper-respiratory infection. For *Pasteurella*—needs to be given at maximum dosage every 4 hours.

Antibiotic	Formulation	Route	Dosage	Comment
'Tylasul Soluble Veterinary' (Elanco)	A soluble powder, each 100 g bottle contains 25 g Tylosin 75 g Sulphathiazole for solution in 40 gallons/190 litres water.	Drinking water.	Use as the only source of water for 3 consecutive days.	Only really applicable to large flocks.
'Tylosin+' (Chevita/Univet)	A soluble powder containing Tylosine Chlortetracycline Arsanilic acid amino acids, vitamins, trace elements in 7.5 g sachets.	Drinking water.	One sachet in 1 litre of drinking water for 3 days.	Formulated for racing pigeons, has been used in parrots and raptors.
Lincomycin				
'Lincocin Sterile Solution' (Upjohn)	A sterile solution for injection containing 100 mg/ml.	i.m.	10–30 mg/kg b.i.d. t.i.d.	A fairly safe antibiotic but apart from its effectiveness against *Mycoplasma* does not have a lot of application to birds. Has been used for skin and feather conditions
'Lincocin Aquadrops' (Upjohn)	Syrup containing 50 mg/ml Supplied with dropper.	Oral.	Budgerigars 1 drop; b.i.d., t.i.d. Amazon parrots 35 mg/300 g; b.i.d., t.i.d. Raptors 175 mg/kg; b.i.d., t.i.d.	(French Moult)—results equivocal. Can cause gastro-intestinal disturbance. Rapidly absorbed, penetrates tissues easily but is rapidly excreted, therefore frequent dosage is necessary.
		Drinking water.	20 drops/100 ml.	

Table 4.7. Antibiotics for use in birds: Chloramphenicol.

Antibiotic	Formulation	Route	Dosage	Comment
'Chloromycetin Succinate' (Parke Davis)	Vial containing 1.2 mg powder for reconstitution in water.	i.m. s.c. i.v.	Large birds 10 – 30 mg/kg, t.i.d. Small birds 80 mg/kg, t.i.d.	A bacteriostatic antibiotic with a wide range of activity against Gram-positive and Gram-negative organisms, *Rickettsia* and some viruses. Has a small non-ionised molecule easily diffusible into all tissues and penetrates cell membranes. Metabolized in the liver and may suppress the immune response and retard wound healing. Rapidly excreted therefore frequent dosage is necessary.
'Ertilen Injection' (Ciba-Geigy) Other formulations available	Stabilized water miscible solution containing 150 mg/ml.	i.m.	50 mg/kg, b.i.d., t.i.d.	
'Chloromycetin Palmitate' (Parke Davis)	An oral suspension containing 30 mg/ml.	Oral.	50 mg/1.6 ml/kg, t.i.d. 0.1 ml/30 g, t.i.d., q.i.d.	
'Chloromycetin Capsules' (Parke Davis)	Each capsule contains a white powder with a 250 mg active ingredient.	Food.	100 – 200 mg/kg.	Can be mixed in food, preferably a mash.
'Ornimed' (L.A.B.)	Canary seed impregnated with 0.1 mg/1 g of Chloramphenicol.	Feed.	1–2 capfuls (1.5 g) per 30 g bird.	Suitable for small birds up to cockatiel in size (100 g). Do not give normal seed until medicated seed is eaten but do not keep normal seed away for more than 10 hours.

Table 4.8. Antibacterial and antiprotozoal drugs: The sulphonamides.
The sulphonamides are active against a wide range of organisms including *Protozoa* and *Rickettsia*. They diffuse widely into all tissues. Only some are well absorbed from the gut. There is some slight danger of precipitation in an acid urine.

Antibiotic	Formulation	Route	Dosage	Comment
Sulphadimidine 'Sulphamezathine' (I.C.I.)	A 1:3 solution sulphadimidine (1 g in 3 ml of water).	Oral Drinking water.	30 ml/4.5 litres for 5 days only or 0.6 ml/100 ml.	Useful for treating coccidiosis.
Combined Sulphonamide 'Ornimed' (L.A.B.)	Canary seed impregnated with Sulphathiazole 0.125 mg Sulphamerazine 0.125 mg Sulphadiazine 0.125 mg Sulphaquinozalium 0.125 mg per 1 g.	Feed.	One capful (1.5 g) per 30 g bird.	Suitable for small birds up to cockatiel in size (100 g).
Trimethoprim combined with Sulphonamides 'Trivetrin'	Stable solution containing.	i.m.	50 mg/kg in psittacines and raptors (of combined active ingredients)	Trimethoprim is lipid soluble and widely

(Wellcome)	Trimethoprim 40 mg; Sulphadoxine 200 mg per 1 ml.	s.c.		distributed in the tissues. Well tolerated with no sign of reaction at the site of injection. Bacteriocidal against Gram-positive and Gram-negative bacteria including *E. coli*, *Pasteurella*, *Proteus*, *Salmonella* and *Listerella*. Inadvisable to administer together with chloramphenicol or the aminoglycosides.
'Septrin Paediatric Suspension' (Wellcome)	A suspension containing Trimethoprim 40 mg Sulphamethoxazole 200 mg in 5 ml.	Oral.	Large birds 100 mg (total active ingredient). Small birds 150 mg (total active ingredient).	
'Tribrissen Oral Suspension' (Wellcome)	A suspension containing Trimethoprim 30 mg Sulphadiazine 400 mg per 1.0 ml.	Drinking water only.	For the treatment of poultry 1 ml/5 litres.	
'Scorprin 120 Capsules' (Willows)	Each capsule contains Trimethoprim 20.0 mg Sulphadiazine 100.0 mg.	Oral or mixed in food.	As for 'Septrin Suspension'.	Open capsule and divide contents.

Table 4.9 (a). Antibacterial and antiprotozoal drugs: the nitrofurazones. The nitrofurazones are active against some Gram-negative bacteria and Coccidia.

Drug	Formulation	Route	Dosage	Comment
Furazolidone 'Coryzium' (Crown)	Capsules containing 20 mg Furazolidone.	Oral.	One capsule per 400 g bird daily for 3 days.	Formulated for the treatment of respiratory conditions in pigeons. Do not overdose—toxic—leads to neurological damage.
'Nifulidone' (Duphar) Other formulations available	A powder dispersible in water containing 5.5% Furazolidone for mixing in pelleted food or drinking water of poultry.	Drinking water.	12.5 – 17.5 g/gallon.	Only really suitable for the treatment of large flocks. Agitate water 4 – 6 times daily.
Furaltadone 'Furasol' (Norwich Eaton)	A soluble powder containing 20% Furaltadone.	Drinking water.	1 kg/1000 litres.	Is used for the treatment of *Salmonella*, coliform and coccidial infections in poultry. Also used to treat sinusitis.

Table 4.9 (b). Drugs are mainly antiprotozal in action.

Drug	Formulation	Route	Dosage	Comment
Dimetriadazole				
'Emtryl' (May & Baker)	Soluble powder containing 40% Dimetriadazole 400 mg/g powder.	Oral in drinking water.	50–100 mg/kg/150 ml drinking water. Daily for 3–5 days. Dissolve 1 heaped teaspoonful in 1.5 pints (840 ml). Give each bird 9.5 ml/30 g.	Toxic if dose is exceeded. Active against trichomoniasis, giardiasis and histomoniasis. Do not use during breeding season. *Do not use in finches—may be toxic.*
			1 oz (30 g) of soluble powder/10 gallons (45 litres).	For the treatment of poultry and game birds.
'Gabbrocol' (Chevita/Univet)	Dimetriadazole, Paromomycine in sachets of 5.0 g.	Drinking water.	One sachet/5.0 g in 2 litres of drinking water 7 – 8 days.	Formulated for racing pigeons.
	In capsules.	Oral.	One capsule per 500 g bird daily 7 – 8 days.	
Metronidazole				
'Flagyl' (May & Baker)	Tablets containing 200 mg Metronidazole.	Oral.	Pigeons one-tenth part of a tablet for 5 days.	Active against *Trichomoniasis* and *Giardiasis.*
'Flagyl-S' (May & Baker)	Suspension containing 200 mg/5ml in a 125 ml bottle.		50 mg/kg once daily.	In humans used against a number of anaerobic infections. Not as toxic as Dimetridazole. *Toxic for finches.*

Table 4.10. Antifungal drugs for use in birds.

Drug	Formulation	Route	Dosage	Comment
Amphotericin sodium 'Fungizone' (Squibb)	A vial containing 50 mg for solution in water for injection.	i.v. Intra-tracheal.	Raptors 1.5 mg/kg, t.i.d. for 3 days. Psittacines and raptors 1 mg/kg, t.i.d. Diluted with water: one vial/100 ml water i.e. 50 mg/100 ml.	Not absorbed from the gut and therefore has to be given by injection. This should be given as slowly as is practical. Active against a wide range of yeast and fungi including *Aspergillus* and *Candida*. Non toxic at the recommended doses. Exceeding the dosage can produce nephrotoxicity and thrombophlebitis. Rapidly excreted.
'Fungilin' (Squibb)	Cream and in orobase.	Topical.	Can be used for lesions in the mouth.	
Nystatin 'Nystan Oral Suspension' (Squibb)	A suspension containing 100,000 units/ in a 30 ml dropper.	Oral.	2–7 ml/kg, b.i.d. or t.i.d. for 7–14 days.	Not absorbed from the gut therefore very safe. Not active against *Aspergillus*. Useful for treating candidiasis.
'Mycostatin-20' (Squibb)	A powder containing 44 g/kg.	In feed.	2.25 kg/20 tonne.	Only suitable for treating large flocks.
Ketoconazole 'Nizoral' (Janssen)	200 mg tablets.	Crop tube or in food.	10 mg/kg.	For treatment of candidiasis. Tablets are not soluble. Found to be highly toxic in a small percentage of humans on long-term dosage about the same may apply to birds.

Drug	Formulation	Route	Dose	Comments
Rifampicin 'Rifadin' (Merrell) 'Rimactane' (Ciba)	Syrup containing 100 mg/5 ml.	Oral.	30 mg/kg, t.i.d.	Active against Gram-positive organisms, mycobacteria and *Aspergillus*. May be hepatoxic.
5-Fluorocystosine 'Alcobon' (Roche)	Tablets containing 500 mg Flucystosine.	Oral.	120 mg–250 mg/kg, in 3 divided dosages Lower doses for large birds.	Active against aspergillosis, fungal and yeast infections. A fairly safe drug at the prescribed doses.
Chlorhexidine 22% 'Hibitane' (I.C.I.)	Hibitane concentrate solution contains 25% Chlorhexidine marketed as an antiseptic.	Drinking water.	10 ml/gallon (USA) (3.8 litres) 12 ml/gallon (imperial) (4.5 litres) 7–14 days.	Consult manufacturer before use. Has been used in the USA for flock treatment of *candidiasis*. Also slows the spread of some viral infections (e.g. *psittacine herpes virus*). May be virucidal. Not absorbed from the gut (Clubb, 1984). used by the author in budgerigars and not found to be toxic at 3 times this dose.
Miconazole 'Daktarin Injection' (Janssen)	Sterile injection containing 10 mg/ml of Miconazole in a 20 ml ampoule.	i.m.	10 mg/kg once daily used in pigeons and raptors (Furley & Greenwood, 1982) in penguins (Gass, 1979).	This dose is safe but equivocal. See Lawrence (1983). Up to 40 mg/kg, i.v. daily is used in children. May be able to give by intratracheal injection.

Table 4.11. Anthelmintics for use in birds.

Anthelmintic	Formulation	Route	Dosage	Comment
Fenbendazole 'Panacure' (Hoechst)	2.5% suspension containing 25 mg/ml. Other formulations are available which might be more useful when treating large numbers of birds.	Oral in feed or by crop tube.	10 – 50 mg/kg daily for 7 days or 100 mg/kg as a single dose. For small birds dilute 1 in 4, then use 0.5 ml/30 g bird.	A broad spectrum anthelmintic with an ovicidal effect on roundworm eggs. Tasteless, odourless, palatable. Can be dropped onto the food or mixed with honey. A safe drug in most species but *must not be used in pigeons—toxic* (Lawrence, 1983).
Mebendazole 'Mebenvet' (Janssen) (Game bird wormer) (Crown Chemical Company)	A powder containing 1.2% active ingredient.	In food.	250 g/25 kg feed use for 7 days. See maker's instructions.	A broad spectrum anthelmintic for use in poultry and game birds. Toxic for Pigeons and Parrots.
Thibendazole 'Thibenzole' (M.S.D.)	Suspension containing 17.6% w/v 176 mg/ml of Thibendazole. Pre-mix containing 25% w/v.	Crop tube or in feed. In feed.	40 – 200 mg/kg once.	Has been used for a variety of birds but is not very efficient since it is only partly active against some nematodes. Ovicidal. *May be toxic for pigeons.* Useful for treating game birds.
Cambendazole 'Ascapilla' (Chevita/Univet)	Capsules containing 30 mg.	Oral.	1 capsule (30 mg)/500 g bird for 2 consecutive days.	Formulated for pigeons. See manufacturer's instructions.

Drug	Preparation	Route	Dose	Notes
Levamisole 'Nemicide' (I.C.I.) Marketed by many other companies	A sterile solution containing 7.5% Levamisole 75 mg/ml.	Oral. Drinking water. i.m.	15–25 mg/kg once Dilute 10–15 times with water. 8 mg/kg.	Active only against nematodes. Has a bitter taste. Withhold drinking water for 8 hours prior to dosing. Do not leave down for more than 24 hours. *Has been given by injection but this is not advisable as it may be toxic in some species in anthelmintic doses—vomiting ataxia.*
'Spartakon' (Crown)	An orange tablet containing the equivalent of 20 mg levamisole.	Oral.	0.1 ml/gallon (4.5 litres).	
		s.c.	2 mg/kg daily for 3 days at 4 day intervals. must be used intermittently.	For immunostimulation in debilitated birds. Has been used in turkeys up to 10 mg/kg for this purpose.
Niclosamide 'Yomesan' (Bayer)	Tablet containing 0.5 g of niclosamide.	Oral. Crop tube. In feed.	250 mg/kg once.	Active against tape worms. Tablets are not soluble. Must be suspended in water or mixed in mash.
Ivermectin 'Ivomec' (M.S.D.)	Sterile solution containing 1% w/v of Ivermectin 10 mg/ml.	i.m.	200 mg/kg once. Dilute 1:9 and use 0.2 ml/kg.	Broad spectrum. Active against *nematodes, tapeworms, Coccidia* and *Knemidokoptes.* Dilute just before use—solution is not stable. Expensive to use.
Piperazine (Vet Drug)	Piperazine Citrate tablets 500 mg.	Oral. Drinking water.	100 mg/kg or 8 g in 1 gallon of drinking water.	Has been used for worming pigeons but is not recommended as it has a narrow margin of safety in some species.

Table 4.12. Agents for use against ectoparasites.

Drug	Formulation	Route	Dosage	Comment
Piperonyl butoxide 'Pybuthrin Dusting Powder' (Vet Drug)	Powder with Piperonyl Butoxide 1.137% w/v, Pyrethrins 0.113% w/v.	External application.	Dust onto feathers.	Safe and effective. Brush out excess from hand held bird.
Derris Powder 'Skin Dressing Derris 2%' (Vet Drug)	Powder containing 2% w/v Derris.	External application.	As above.	As above.
Bromocyclen 'Alugan' (Hoechst)	(1) Sachet containing 20 g.	External application.	1 sachet of 20 g in 2 gallons (9 litres) of water to make 0.2% solution	Active against all external parasites. Apply to head and legs for mange mites.
	(2) Dusting powder.	External application.	Dust into feathers.	Dust out excess powder.
Coumaphos 'Negasunt' (Bayer)	Powder containing 3% w/v Coumaphos, 2% w/v Propxur, 5% w/v Sulphanilamide.	External application.	Dust into plumage.	Active against all external parasites. Useful for fly blown wounds.

Gamma benzine hexachloride			
Contained in various canine aural preparations.		External application.	Applied *very* sparingly to head and legs and make sure none is inhaled or swallowed.
'Auroid' (Willows)	0.10% w/v BHC and antibiotics.		Although the chlorinated hydrocarbons are considered to be toxic for birds all the preparations have been used by the author at one time or another for the treatment of *Knemidocoptic mange* without toxic effects.
'GA.C. Ear Drops' (Dales)	0.10% w/v BHC and antibiotics.		
Griseofulvin			
'Fulcin' (I.C.I.)	Tablets containing 125 mg of Griseofulvin.	Oral.	No recommended dose.
'Grisovin' (Glaxo)			Active against *Trichophyton* species. No action against *Aspergillus* or *Candida*.

Table 4.13. Hormones for use in birds.

Hormone	Formulation	Route	Dosage	Comment
Testosterone 'Androject' (Intervet)	An oily solution for injection containing 10 mg Testosterone Phenylpropionate per ml.	i.m. s.c.	2 – 6 mg/kg once 2.5 mg/kg weekly for 6 weeks.	For stimulation of sexual behaviour in the male. Has been used for baldness in the canary. Should not be used in birds with liver disease.
'Duratestone' (Intervet)	An oily solution for injection containing 4 esters of testosterone 50 mg total esters/ml.	i.m. s.c.	50 mg/kg once.	Prolonged activity over 2 weeks.
Testosterone implants (Intervet)	A white opaque sterile cylinder containing 25 mg of testosterone.	s.c.	One 25 mg implant/kg.	Prolonged activity over 4 – 5 weeks.
Nandrolone cyclohexyl proprionate 'Retarbolin' (Berk)	Sterile oily injection containing 10 mg/ml.	i.m.	0.4 mg/kg. once 0.02 mg/30 g.	Chronic and debilitating disease. Should not be used if there is liver disease.
Dexamethosone 'Dexadreson' (Intervet)	A clear aqueous solution containing 2 mg/ml.	i.m. Topically	0.3 – 3 mg/kg Mixed in 50% solution with D.S.M.O.	To reduce the inflammatory response and combat shock. Preferably given with appropriate antibiotics.

Drug	Preparation	Route	Dose	Indication
Delmadinone 'Tardak' (Syntex)	An aqueous suspension containing 10 mg/ml.	i.m.	1 mg/kg. 0.02 ml/30 g. once	Neurotic regurgitation in budgerigars—sometimes effective. Well tolerated.
Medroxyprogesterone 'Promone-E' (Upjohn) 'Perlutex' (Leo)	Aqueous suspension containing 50 mg/ml. Aqueous suspension containing 28 mg/ml.	i.m.	30 mg/kg.	Neurotic regurgitation in budgerigars. Also some feather conditions involving excess preening. Has been used for persistant egg laying in budgerigars.
Oxytocin 'Oxytocin-S' (Intervet)	A clear aqueous solution containing 10 units/ml.	i.m.	0.3 – 0.5 ml/kg.	Used in conjunction with calcium borogluconate for impaction of the oviduct. See Chapter 6, p. 142.
Atropine 'Atropine Sulpate' (Vet Drug)	A sterile solution for injection containing 600 mcg/ml 0.6 mg/ml.	i.m. s.c.	0.05–0.1 mg/kg, 0.1–0.6 ml/kg use higher doses for small birds only.	For premedication 10 minutes prior to anaesthesia. As a partial antidote to organophosphorous poisoning.
(Bimeda)	A solution containing 10 mg/ml.			
Thyroxine 'Eltroxine' (Glaxo)	Tablets containing 0.05 mg.	In drinking water.	0.025 mg ($\frac{1}{2}$–$\frac{3}{4}$ tablet) 100 ml for 4 weeks.	Hypothyroidism. Double the dose for birds that drink little. The tablets are not very soluble.
		Oral.	Up to .1 mg/kg.	To induce moult—use only for 7 days.

Table 4.14. Miscellaneous drugs for use in birds.

Drug	Formulation	Route	Dosage	Comment
Iodine 'Lugols iodine'	Lugols iodine B.P.	In drinking water.	Dilute by adding 2 parts to 28 parts of water. Add 3 drops of this solution to 100 ml drinking water—use for 3 weeks.	Secondary thyroid hyperplasia due to iodine deficiency commonly seen in budgerigars.
Sodium iodide	20% sterile solution for injection 200 mg/ml.	i.m.	0.01 – 0.03 ml(2 mg – 6 mg)/30g bird 0.33 – 1.0 ml(66 – 133 mg)/kg body weight.	Secondary thyroid hyperplasia due to iodine deficiency. Considerable improvement to respiratory obstruction seen within 3 days.
Potassium iodide		In drinking water.	100 – 200 mg/100 ml.	As a palliative in the treatment of chronic respiratory disease. Should not be given for periods longer than a week.
Bromhexidine 'Bisolvon' (Boehringer)	Sterile solution for injection containing 3 mg/ml Bromhexine Hydrochloride. Tablet containing 8 mg (Medical Product).	i.m.	3–6 mg/(1–2 ml)/kg, 0.1 ml/30 g divided into 2 or 3 doses daily.	May help better penetration of the antibiotics and gamma globulins into respiratory tract. Well tolerated. The injection is water-based so can be given orally or in daily water intake (Ahlers, 1970).

Drug	Preparation	Route	Dose	Indications
Allopurinol 'Zyloric' (Calmic) (Wellcome) 'Aluline' (Steinhard)	100 mg tablet.	Oral. Drinking water.	40 mg/kg., Crush a 100 mg tablet. Mix in 10 ml water. Use 2.6 ml of this solution to 100 ml. Give daily for life.	Treatment of gout. Reduces the level of uric acid in the plasma by reducing its production in the liver i.e. inhibits xanthine oxidase which catalyses purines to uric acid.
Calcium Borogluconate	10%(100 mg) ml.	i.v. s.c.	1–5 ml (100–500 mg) per kg, by *slow* intravenous injection.	Treatment of impaction of the oviduct and egg binding used *together with* oxytocin. Treatment of raptors with 'fits' due to hypocalcaemia. Advisable to give Dextrose injection at the same time.

Table 4.15 (a) Vitamins and nutritional supplements.

Drug	Formulation	Route	Dosage	Comment
Multivitamin and mineral				
'S.A. 37' (Intervet) 'Vionate' (Squibb)	See maker's data and information sheets.	Oral.	500 mg/kg.	May be wasteful when mixed with seed. Needs to be given in a mash.
Multivitamin Injections (C-Vet) (Pharmavet)	See maker's date and information sheets.	i.m.	0.5 ml/kg supplying 7,500 i.u. vitamin A and other vitamins.	Vitamin A overdose is toxic and can produce skeletal abnormalities and damage to membranes.
Multivitamin Drops 'Abidec' (Parke Davis)	See makers' data and information sheets. Vitamin A approx/6,500 units/ml.	Drinking water.	5 drops/0.3 ml/30 g bird, every third day.	
'Vitin' (Chevita/Univet)	Vitamins, trace elements, minerals, amino acids, sugars and fatty acids 100 ml bottles.	Oral. Drinking water.	2–3 drops/30 g. 3–5 drops/pigeons.	Metabolic support in stress and conditions associated with infectious disease.
'Multivitamin +' (Chevita/Univet)	Sachets containing 8.0 g of 12 vitamins, trace elements and Methenamine.	In drinking water.	One sachet/5 litres.	
'Ornimed' Vit B$_{12}$ (L.A.B.)	Canary impregnated seed containing vitamin B$_{12}$ 4 mcg/g.	Oral.	1.5 g (one capfull)/30 bird.	For the treatment of reduced hatchability and retarded growth.
'Duphalyte' (Duphar)	An injectable solution of electrolytes, vitamins amino acids and dextrose.	s.c. i.v.	10 ml/kg, b.i.d.	Given in the groin or at base of neck with Hyaluronidase. Give *very slowly* i.v.

Table 4.15 (b) Minerals and nutritional supplements.

Drug	Formulation	Route	Dosage	Comment
'Lamb Tonic' (Crown)	A liquid containing 18 amino acids, 10 B vitamins, glucose and sugars in 30 ml bottles.	Oral.	10 ml/kg.	Supportive therapy.
'Ovigest Elixir' (Wellcome)	A sterile liquid containing 8% protein digest 10% glucose w/v 100 ml containers.	Oral.	10ml/kg.	Support therapy. Discard if liquid becomes cloudy.
Natural Yoghurt	Contains *Lactobacillus acidophilus*.	Oral.	2 ml/kg.	May help to restore gut flora after antibiotic therapy. Controversial but will do no harm.
Invalid Foods 'Farlene' (Farley Health Foods) 'Complan' (Carnation Foods) 'Build Up' 'Vita Food' (Boots Ltd.)	Human invalid foods that contain approx. 4 calories/g of food.	By crop tube.	100 g/kg daily. 7.5 g/30 g daily.	Best results obtained in the severely debilitated bird by dividing daily dose and giving at hourly intervals.
'Collovet' (C-Vet)	A liquid containing iron, copper, manganese, chromium, caffeine, thiamine and glycerophosphates.	Oral. In drinking water.	1 – 2 drops (0.06–0.12 ml)/30 g bird in drinking water every other day.	General tonic to stimulate appetite in anorexia and debility.
'Vi-Sorbin' (Smith Kline)	A liquid containing cyanocobalamin 834 mcg Vit B_6, 2 mg, ferric-pyrophosphate 100 mg, folic acid 0.5 mg, sorbitol 4.4 ml/5 ml.	Oral.	0.6 ml/kg.	As above for collovet.

Table 4.16. drugs acting on the alimentary canal.

Drug	Formulation	Route	Dosage	Comment
Liquid Paraffin Mineral Oil		Oral per cloacum.	4 ml/kg.	For impaction of the cloaca and egg binding.
Glycerine		Oral per cloacum.	5 ml/kg.	
Sucrose in water	30% solution.	Oral.	up to 10 ml/kg.	Mild purgative.
Antidiarrhoeals without antibiotic. **Kaolin mixtures**				*Antidiarrhoeals without antibiotic.*
B.P.C. (Vet Drug)	Light kaolin B.P. 20% w/v **Light magnesium carbonate 5% w/v** Sodium bicarbonate B.P. 5% w/v			
'Stat' (Intervet)	Light kaolin 10.8 g Aluminium hydroxide gel 1.93 g Sodium acetate 1.98 g Sodium chloride 1.8 lg. Potassium acetate 330 mg Magnesium chloride 100 mg Calcium chloride 100 mg in each 100 ml.	Oral.	3 ml/kg, b.i.d., t.i.d.	Note many birds that are anorexic have watery droppings but do not have diarrhoea.

'Kaogel' (Parke Davis)	Light kaolin 3 g Pectin 65 mg in 15 ml.			
Kaopectate (Upjohn)	Kaolin 1.03 g in 5 ml.			

Antidiarrhoels with neomycin and/or some sulphonamide.

'Kaobiotic Suspension' (Upjohn)	Neomycin sulphate 229 mg Sulphaquanidine 6.87 mg Sulphamerazine 415 mg Sulphadiazine 415 mg Sulphathiazole 415 mg Pectin 750 mg Kaolin 20.5 mg in each 100 ml	Oral.	1 ml – 1.5 ml/kg t.i.d.	Do not overdose because of absorption of some of the sulphonamide, and kidney may already be compromised in diarrhoea cases.
'Nuvamide' Suspension (May & Baker)	Sulphadiazine 25 mg Sulphapyradine 25 mg Sulphamerazine 25 mg Neomycin sulphate 17.86 mg Light Kaolin 160 mg in each one ml.			

Table 4.17. Sedatives and stimulant drugs.

Drug	Formulation	Route	Dosage	Comment
Diazepam 'Valium' (Roche)	Ampoules containing 10 mg/2 ml.	i.m.	10 mg/kg.	These doses are sedative doses. For anaesthetic doses see Chapter 5.
Ketamin 'Vetalar' (Parke Davis)	Sterile solution for injection containing 100 mg/ml.	i.m.	Up to 15 mg/kg.	Not very reliable as sedatives.
Xylazine 'Rompun' (Bayer)	Sterile aqueous solution for injection 20 mg/ml.	i.m.	Up to 2 mg/kg.	
Reserpine 'Sermix' (Ciba-Geigy)	A powder containing 0.2% w/v (2 mg/g) reserpine.	In feed.	2 – 4 mg/kg in meat for raptors; 5 – 6 days tranquilization stops them eating so that they have to be force-fed. 8 g/15 kg feed for game birds (Green, 1979). 0.0625 g/ton of feed for tranquilization of geese (Wilgus, 1960). 1 kg/11 tons of turkey feed.	Marketed for use in turkeys. Lowers blood pressure and reduces chances of aortic rupture due to aneurysm. Also has a marked sedative effect.

Doxapram hydrochloride				
'Dopram-V' (A.H. Robins)	Multidose vials containing 20 mg/ml Doxapram Hydrochloride.	Oral. i.m.	**One drop in a small bird's mouth.** 7 mg/kg (0.3 ml/kg) 0.01 mg/30 g.	Respiratory stimulant when apnoea occurs. To stimulate breathing in newly hatched chicks.
Respirot (Ciba)	A syrup containing Crotethamide 75 mg/ml. Cropropamide 75 mg/ml.	Oral.	One drop in the mouth of a pigeon-sized bird 2 drops/kg.	Do not use in small birds below 100 g.
Sodium Calciumedetate				
B. Vet C. (Vet Drug)	A sterile solution containing 25% w/v 250 mg/ml.	i.v. i.m. s.c.	62.5 mg (0.25 ml) kg for swans given s.c., t.i.d. (Cooke, 1984)	For lead poisoning. If given i.v. give slowly, s.c. may cause some slight reaction.
'Ledclair' (Sinclair)	Contains 200 mg/ml.		May be able to increase dose to 80 – 100 mg/kg for smaller birds.	May need to give for prolonged periods up to six weeks.

5 / Anaesthesia

General considerations

Before selecting an anaesthetic the practitioner should take into account the reasons for its use.

Hypnosis and restraint

Perhaps the main indication for using an anaesthetic drug is to produce chemical restraint whilst radiography is carried out or endoscopy or some other non-painful procedure is performed. There are a number of drugs or combinations of injectable agents suitable for the purpose but which have little analgesic effect.

Analgesia

The abolition of painful stimuli may be the prime consideration. If this is to produce analgesia of a limited surface area then local anaesthetics can be used. These have not been very popular with many clinicians in the past, particularly the drugs of the procaine-based group which have a reputation for toxicity. This is most probably because many small birds were grossly overdosed. Local anaesthetics are safe in birds if the dose is carefully calculated.

Some operations on poultry such as the relief of an impacted crop or ovarectomy have in the past been carried out without any anaesthetic and with little apparent distress to the bird. There is little doubt that the level of sensory perception is low in many parts of the avian skin. Cutting the integument seems to provoke much less response than stretching or undermining the skin. Those parts of the bird's anatomy that are most sensitive are the cere, the comb, the wattles, the cloaca and the surrounding skin, the scaled parts of the legs and the pads of the feet. However, there is some individual and interspecies variation in the tenderness of the feet, particularly in raptors.

Muscle relaxation

This may be required during surgery, particularly orthopaedic surgery when there is often contracture of muscle groups around a fracture site. Some anaesthetic agents, although good hypnotics, do not relax muscle.

The relief of anxiety and fear for the patient

Although placed last on this list, it is by no means the least important consideration. Anxiety and fear by the bird considerably increase stress and reduce the chances of survival after an operation. It is for this reason that an anaesthetic technique may be chosen which goes some way in combining all the above-mentioned requirements of anaesthesia and that can only be achieved using a balanced combination of drugs.

Assessment of the avian patient for anaesthesia

The clinician should be aware that there is not only an interspecies disparity in the response of birds to a particular anaesthetic agent but there is also some individual variation. This is probably due to differences in liver and plasma enzymes systems and the rate of detoxication and excretion of the anaesthetic. This is more evident than is the case in related mammalian species. The bird that panics when handled or is difficult to catch will have an increased adrenaline outflow and will cause anxiety during anaesthesia. Conversely, the bird that is too easily caught and is just picked off its perch is also a worry. Wild birds are normally frightened or aggressive; if they are not, they are ill. It is better to delay anaesthesia in this group of patients for 48 hours so that they have a chance to feed and reach a better nutritional status.

A falcon in flying condition or a racing pigeon is usually athletically fit. However, many falconers keep their birds hungry to make them keen hunters. If the bird becomes sick it may be very near hypoglycaemia with depleted liver glycogen reserves.

An aged parrot (it is not uncommon to see one that is 35–40 years old) may have spent most of its life in a cage and may be obese or have atheromatous arteries. Small birds kept in aviaries are more likely to be fit than their caged fellows. A bird that is chronically ill or suffering from a low-grade toxaemia will have a depressed rate of detoxication of drugs.

Because of all these factors, always carry out a clinical assessment of the patient before giving the anaesthetic. Take a blood sample and do a microhaematocrit. If the PCV is over 55% the bird needs rehydrating with fluid therapy as described in Chapter 7, p. 173. If the PCV is below 20%, then theoretically, the bird needs blood. If a donor pigeon is available blood from this bird can be given on a once-only basis to any species. Subsequent transfusions will produce a reaction (p. 125). For an indication of the quantity that can be given see p. 20. If a refractometer is available carry out a total serum protein evaluation, which will give an indication of the nutritional status of the bird.

Theoretically it would be better to determine the albumin/globulin ratio but as (Galvin, 1978) has indicated, the largest portion of serum protein is albumin and a reduction in serum protein is usually caused by a drop in albumen levels, rather than a fall in the globulins.

Some physiological considerations

The avian lung compared to that in a mammal of comparable size is small and non-expansible. The evolution of the fixed-volume avian lung has taken place along with the development of a rigid meshwork of blood and air capillaries. The largest diameter of the air capillaries of birds being less than one-third the size of the smallest mammalian alveoli. The very small diameter of the non-collapsible terminal airway, produces a high pressure gradient for the diffusion of blood gases (King and McLelland, 1984b). The system provides a greatly increased gaseous exchange surface—about 10 times that in a mammal of comparable body weight. The blood flow in the lung in relation to the air flow is principally cross-current. In the mammal the blood and gas flows are more linear. This again increases the efficiency of gas exchange in the avian lung.

The air sacs take no part in gaseous exchange and act merely as bellows driving the air in a one way flow through the respiratory tract, as illustrated in Fig. 5.1. The air sacs do however greatly increase the dead space (approximately 34% in the chicken). Because of this unidirectional air flow in the avian lung, inhaled anaesthetic gases go first to the posterior air sacs before any gas exchange takes place, and are then passed through the lung before being exhaled via the anterior air sacs. If apnoea ensues because too much anaesthetic gas has been administered, and artificial respiration has to be started, then further absorbtion of anaesthetic gas will take place as it passes through the lung exchange surface

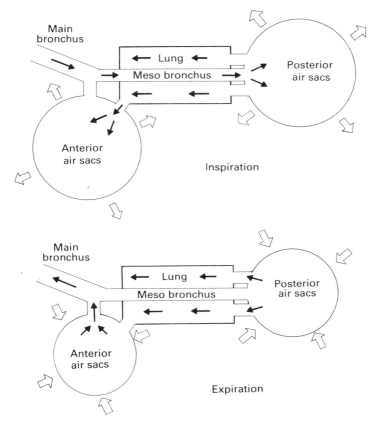

Fig. 5.1. Diagrammatic representation of the function of the avian respiratory system illustrating the uniflow of gas through the exchange surface of the lung.

from that stored in the posterior air sacs. The net effect of the anatomy and physiology of the avian respiratory system is to make gaseous exchange much more rapid and efficient than in the mammal. Volatile anaesthetics can reach dangerous plasma concentrations very quickly.

Another physiological aspect of the rigid lung is that the chemo receptors monitoring $PaCO_2$ are much more important than the mechano receptors monitoring pressure changes (Fedde & Kuhlman, 1977). The $PaCO_2$ of the domestic fowl is normally about 30% lower than in mammals because of the more efficient 'washout' in the avian lung. Birds are thus much more sensitive to hypercapnia.

It is therefore important to maintain high gas flow rates of oxygen during avian anaesthesia. These should be at least three times the normal minute volume. Klide (1973) gives the following normal minute volumes:

(1)   domestic fowl weighing 2.5 kg, the minute volume is 770 ml/minute;

(2)   racing pigeon weighing about 300 g, the minute volume is 250 ml/minute;

(3)   a small cage bird weighing 30 g, the minute volume is 25 ml/minute.

In practice the author uses flow rates of not less than 0.7 litres/ minute for the small birds and 3 litres per minute for birds the size of domestic fowl.

Marley & Payne (1964) demonstrated when using halothane anaesthesia that the $PaCO_2$ gradually increased during prolonged anaesthesia even in those birds where respiration appeared to be normal. In birds where respiration was depressed the $PaCO_2$ increased much more rapidly (from 18–27 mm Hg to 50–75 mm Hg within 10 minutes). If the $PaCO_2$ rose to 80 mm Hg the bird died.

King & Payne (1964) showed that in the chicken, when the bird was placed in dorsal recumbency the minute volume could be reduced by a factor of 10–60%. This was brought about by the pressure on the air sacs by the viscera. These workers showed that the effect was greater in the female than in the male and was less if the bird was in lateral recumbency.

The effects of hypoxia vary in different groups of birds. Nevertheless the oxygen uptake is higher in all birds than in mammals of comparable size. High-flying birds and diving ducks can withstand the effects of oxygen withdrawal better than surface-feeding ducks and birds that are mainly terrestrial (Dawson, 1975). The Gentoo and Chinstrap penguin, which remain submerged for long periods, withstand hypoxia better than the Adélie penguin which is a short-term diver.

Many agents used in general anaesthesia are also respiratory depressants. All these factors make the maintenance of an adequate rate of respiration together with relatively high flow rates of oxygen very important, whatever type of anaesthetic technique is being used. Failing this, the $PaCO_2$ can build up rapidly and without warning. Even if there is a high flow rate of oxygen, the elimination of carbon dioxide may be inefficient. If the bird's respiratory rate is allowed to drop to a level where it is just perceptible it may be irreversible. A condition of respiratory acidosis quickly supervenes, the myocardium is depressed and blood pressure drops. A raised $PaCO_2$ predisposes to atrial and ventricular fibrillation and to cardiac failure.

Hypothermia, which affects all birds under anaesthesia particularly the small ones, also helps to depress the myocardium.

Because of the large internal surface area of the air sacs, there may be a high fluid loss during prolonged anaesthesia. In an already dehydrated bird this could be critical and lead to a reduced circulating blood volume with a fall in cardiac output, reduced tissue perfusion and to anaerobic respiration. This in turn leads to a fall in plasma pH and a condition of metabolic acidosis ensues. Many anaesthetics also depress blood pressure.

Cardiac failure during anaesthesia of birds is most likely to be caused by hypocapnia, but hypoxia, the anaesthetic agent, dehydration, hypothermia and the positioning of the patient are all contributing factors.

Suggested precautionary measures during general anaesthesia of avian patients

(1) Whether employing an injectable or volatile anaesthetic agent always administer oxygen. Preferably have an endotracheal tube in place to maintain a clear airway and to enable artificial ventilation, should this prove necessary.

(2) It is safer to have too high a rate of flow of oxygen than one that is too low.

(3) Make sure the respiratory rate is not reduced too much and maintain as light a plane of anaesthesia as is possible.

(4) If possible use lateral or sternal recumbency.

(5) Use a heat pad and do not make the bird too wet during pre-operation preparation. Keep the table top dry. Maintain a comfortable high operating room ambient temperature. If there is a forced air ventilation system, reduce any air currents to a minimum.

(6) Green (1979) suggests leaving a long piece of capillary tubing, with the tip in the oropharynx of a very small bird, to aspirate any excess mucus by capillary action.

(7) It is useful to have a syringe with an attached piece of catheter ready, in case it is necessary to aspirate any mucus blocking the airway.

(8) Premedicate the bird with atropine. Atropine may reduce excess respiratory secretions and it will also reduce any tendency to bradycardia induced by vagal stimulation through traction on the viscera. It should be noted that Cooper (1974) found that atropine did not reduce mucus secretion caused when using metomidate. Atropine may also help reduce contraction of the smooth muscle in the meso- and parabronchi, which in turn reduces gaseous exchange.

Some workers (Marley & Payne, 1964) consider the use of atropine equivocal. However, there can be very few anaesthetic situations where atropine does harm and it may be beneficial.

(9) Do not stretch the wings out too tightly. There may be damage and stimulation to the nerves of the brachial plexus. In addition if the bird is in light anaesthesia and the anaesthetic agent does not give complete muscle relaxation of the pectoralis muscles, movement of the thorax may be restricted.

(10) Use fluid therapy if the bird is anaesthetized for any period longer than 20 minutes. Use 0.1 ml of Ringer lactate intramuscularly for a 30 g budgerigar, every 10 minutes or 5 ml/kg/hour for larger birds. This is particularly important if the anaesthetic drug is excreted through the kidneys. The addition of glucose to the Ringer lactate solution helps the liver detoxicate drugs.

(11) Where practical, monitor the avian patient. An oesophageal stethoscope is easy to insert—an oscilloscope is better. A declining heart rate usually means deepening anaesthesia. Using an 'Imp' respiratory monitor (Imp Electronics) gives reassurance.

An indwelling electronic thermometer is also a useful aid.

(12) For birds weighing more than one kg withold food for 12 hours prior to anaesthesia. For those between 300 g–1 kg withold food for 6 hours, between 100–300 g withhold food for 3–4 hours. *Bird below 100 g do not withhold food at all.*

Local anaesthesia

2% Lignocaine hydrochloride with adrenaline

This is quite safe in all but very small birds which are easily over-dosed. For a 30 g bird 0.3 ml would be fatal. It is always safer to dilute the 2% solution to produce a 0.5% solution and the injection should always include adrenaline to limit the rate of absorbtion. In birds over 2 kg, 1–3 ml can safely be used and in a pigeon-sized bird (400 g) up to 1 ml can be used. For surface anaesthesia of the glottis prior to endotracheal entubation, the author regularly uses 1–2 drops approximately 1.5 mg of lignocaine directly on the mucosa. Lignocaine ointment may be useful around the vent after a cloacal prolapse.

2% Procaine hydrochloride

This has been used in the larger birds without difficulty but care needs to be exercised with the dosage because of the drug's narrow safety margin. Again the 2% preparation is best diluted to produce a 0.2% solution when 1–2 ml/kg can safely be used.

0.5% Proparacaine hydrochloride*

This is a useful surface anaesthetic which can be used on the cornea, on the mucosa of the glottis and on the cloaca. One drop is usually sufficient and more than two drops should not be used because this can be toxic.

General anaesthesia

Pre-anaesthetic medication and tranquillization

As mentioned earlier, always use atropine. There are very few general anaesthetic techniques that are not improved with atropine.

The use of tranquillizing drugs such as acetylpromazine has very little effect. Both methohexitone[†] and metomidate[‡] have been used for sedating birds. In the case of the metomidate this is mixed with grain or other food at the rate of 2 g/30 g of food. The drug in solution is mixed with the food and allowed to dry. Sedation occurs in about 10 minutes providing the birds eat all the food. The method is not very reliable.

Some of the injectable anaesthetic agents mentioned below, which are not in themselves entirely satisfactory anaesthetics, make very good hypnotic or induction anaesthetics. These can then be supplemented with volatile anaesthetics so that the desired depth of anaesthesia can be achieved.

---

* 'Ophthaine' (Squibb).
[†] 'Brietal sodium' (Elanco Products Co. Ltd).
[‡] 'Hypnodil' [Janssen Pharmaceutica (C Rown Chemical Co.)].

Assessment of the depth of general anaesthesia

This can be difficult and although it is convenient to classify general anaesthesia into light, medium and deep planes, the response of the individual bird to the stimulation of various reflexes shows considerable variation. Sometimes a bird that is apparently deeply asleep will be awoken suddenly by the stimulation of a particularly sensitive area. The skillful clinician relies on his experience and knowledge of a particular anaesthetic technique and the response of the species on which it is being used. He will primarily observe the depth, rate and pattern of respiration, noting any sudden changes. The aim should be to maintain the patient in light- to medium- depth anaesthesia in which the response to stimulation of the cere, the wattles, the comb and the cloaca together with the surrounding skin is *just* abolished or is sluggish. Pinching the interdigital web of the foot or the undersurface of the foot produces a variable and unreliable response, particularly in raptors. The eyelids may be closed but the corneal reflex, indicated by the nictitating membrane sliding obliquely across the eye, should be sluggish but never entirely lost. If there is no corneal reflex the bird is too deep. Obviously if righting reflexes are not completely abolished the plane of anaesthesia is too light. Respiration should be regular not too slow (not much less than half the normal resting respiratory rate) and deep. A rapid, shallow or intermittent respiration indicates the depth of anaesthesia is too great.

Injectable general anaesthetics

Alphaxalone–Alphadolone*

This drug has been used widely both by intravenous and intramuscular injection—also intraperitoneally. When given intravenously induction is rapid and anaesthesia lasts for about 10 minutes, with good muscle relaxation. When first given there is a fall in blood pressure and there is some respiratory depression. The drug is safe for most raptors when given at the rate of 10 mg/kg i.v. (Cooper, 1978) and has been used in dosages as high as 36 mg/kg i.v. (Harcourt-Brown, 1978). However, Cooper & Redig (1975) experienced cardiac irregularities and deaths when using it on Red-Tailed Hawks and Cribb & Haig (1977) demonstrated serious cardiac irregularities

* 'Saffan' (Glaxovet).

in Red-Tailed Hawks and waterfowl. Haig (1980) also showed that there was a temporary apnoea lasting approximately 46 seconds after intravenous injection.

It can be used in small birds by intraperitoneal injection at the rate of 55 mg/kg when it will sedate the bird. Samour *et al.* (1984) considered it to be the injectable drug of choice for *cranes, flamingoes, storks, turacos, vultures and hornbills.*

The drug has been used in parrots. It is not a really effective anaesthetic unless used intravenously. Because of the fragility of avian veins and the risk of haematoma formation in a struggling bird, intravenous injection is only practical in a moderately sized bird.

With the exception of the above species mentioned by Samour, the author considers that this drug has no advantages over ketamine and its various combinations. There is also the increased risk of heart failure if the heart is not healthy.

Pentobarbitone sodium

This has been used successfully by a number of workers. At the rate of 30–40 mg/kg intravenously it was used by Graham Jones (1966) in pigeons and by Hill & Noakes (1964) in fowls. Delius (1966) used it in gulls intramuscularly at the rate of 80 mg/kg. Sykes (1964) gave 0.3–0.5 ml by rapid intravenous injection to fowls weighing between 2–4 kg and followed this by 0.5 – 1 ml given more slowly until required depth of anaesthesia was reached.

Thiopentone Sodium

The author has used this successfully intravenously in swans at the rate of 30 mg/kg. Sykes (1964) used it in chickens at the rate of 50 mg/kg.

The margin of safety with both pentobarbitone sodium and thiopentone sodium is rather narrow.

Equithesin

This is a mixture of pentobarbitone, chloral hydrate and magnesium sulphate which is used intramuscularly. It gives reasonably good anaesthesia with a reasonable safety margin but is not obtainable commercially.

*Methohexitone Sodium**

Has been given by rapid intravenous injection at the rate of 4–8 mg/kg. Anaesthesia lasts 4–5 minutes (Green, 1979).

Metomidate[†]

This is one of the safest drugs to use on birds with a wide margin of safety. At a dose of 10 – 15 mg/kg intramuscularly it produces hypnosis with good muscle relaxation in about 3 – 5 minutes but it is not a good analgesic. The hypnosis lasts 5 – 15 minutes. The drug has no effect on the cardiovascular system. Some birds such as pigeons, penguins and some ducks may require higher doses. It is not satisfactory in *Ciconiiformes* (storks and cranes) in which it produces marked excitement during recovery (Jones, 1977). Cooper (1970, 1974) has used it at the rate of 5 – 15 mg/kg intramuscularly and has obtained deep anaesthesia in some individual raptors.

Camburn & Stead (1966, 1967) were not confident that true anaesthesia was ever attained when using the drug on wild birds. The author has used it on a number of species and found that in most cases there is a tendency for wing flapping to occur in both the induction and recovery stages.

Xylazine[‡]

When used by itself in doses of 10 mg/kg intramuscularly it produces narcosis but not true anaesthesia. However, it is not a very satisfactory anaesthetic or hypnotic agent. Not only is recovery time prolonged but there is nearly always excitement and even severe convulsions during induction in some species. It can cause bradycardia and partial atrioventricular heart block, there is decreased respiration and often muscle tremors. Although the fatal dose is approximately ten times the therapeutic dose it is not a particularly safe drug to use by itself.

It is not satisfactory at all in the domestic fowl even in doses as high as 100 mg/kg (Green & Simpkin 1984).

Ketamine

This dissociative anaesthetic produces a cataleptic state and has been

---

* 'Brietal Sodium' (Elanco products).
† 'Hypodil' (Janssen Pharmaceutica).
‡ 'Rompun' (Bayer).

widely used in birds both by itself and in combination with synergistic drugs. It has no analgesic effect.

In almost all species when given intramuscularly it produces anaesthesia in approximately 3–5 minutes. Incoordination, opisthotony and relaxation are evident within 1 – 3 minutes of the injection and anaesthesia lasts about 35 minutes. The eyes may or may not remain open. A palpebral reflex is present and muscle relaxation is not very good. There may be some excitement during recovery. The blood pressure and heart rate are slightly lowered and there is some respiratory depression.

Mandelker (1973) used it in budgerigars and other birds at doses ranging from 50 – 100 mg/kg. The author has used it in the budgerigar at a dose of 50 mg/kg for anaesthesia on three consecutive days without ill effect. Green (1979) uses it at 15 mg/kg for induction of anaesthesia which he maintains on 0.5 – 1.0% halothane in 50% nitrous oxide.

Altman (1980) suggests it has an adverse effect on the thermo regulatory centre in some species.

For raptors it has been used in doses ranging from 2.5 mg – 170 mg/kg.

Ketamine is broken down by the liver and excreted by the kidney so that it is important that fluid therapy is used if there is any doubt about the bird being dehydrated.

Ketamine and Acetyl Promazine

Both Stunkard & Miller (1974) and Steiner & Davis (1981) have used this drug combination stating that there is a smoother recovery with less wing flapping than with ketamine alone. The workers use one millilitre of acetyl/promazine containing 20 mg* added to a 10 ml vial of ketamine containing 100 mg/ml. The dose of ketamine is then calculated at 25–50 mg/kg without taking into account the acetyl promazine in the vial. The bird is therefore receiving a dose of acetyl promazine of 0.5–1.0 mg/kg.

Ketamine and Metomidate

This has been used at the rate of 15 mg/kg ketamine together with 40

---

* Acepromazine maleate B.P.C. contains 10 mg/ml for large animals and 2 mg/ml for small animals.

mg/kg metomidate. It produced deep sedation with muscle relaxation in Galliformes (Green & Simpkin 1984).

Ketamine and Diazepam

Redig & Duke (1976) used 20–40 mg/kg of ketamine together with 1.0–1.5 mg/kg of diazepam. Forbes (1984) and Lawton (1984) also report using this combination at the same dose rate given intramuscularly. The combined drugs have been used on Psittacines, Galliformes, Anseriformes, Passeriformes and raptors and the results were generally good with deep sedation or anaesthesia and good muscle relaxation. However Forbes reported that recovery was prolonged in raptors. Both drugs have some depressant effect on respiration.

Ketamine and Xylazine

This combination produces safe hypnosis or anaesthesia in a wide range of species. Muscle relaxation is fairly good and respiration is only slightly depressed. The eyes are sometimes closed and the palpebral reflex is sluggish or absent. The depth, the duration and the length of the recovery time to some degree depend on the dose of ketamine used. The combination has been used in various ratios of the two drugs. Increasing the amount of xylazine in relation to the ketamine has very little beneficial effect since the main effect of the xylazine appears to be to reduce the rate of breakdown of the ketamine. Redig (1983) has two routines when using this combination on raptors.

(1)   Three-quarters of the computed dose is given rapidly intravenously; one minute is allowed to assess the effect; then the rest of the dose is given slowly.

(2)   Alternatively, three-quarters of the dose may be given intramuscularly then if necessary the rest of the dose intravenously but to effect. If this does not produce sufficient relaxation and there is still some wing flapping a further one-half the original computed dose is given. Redig (1983) and also Haigh (1980) found that when this drug combination was given intravenously there were some cardiac irregularities and disturbance of the respiratory pattern. This does not happen if the combination is used intramuscularly. Haigh at first used a dose intravenously of 30–40 mg/kg of ketamine together with 0.5 – 1.0 mg/kg of xylazine. This worker now uses a dose of 2.5 – 5.0 mg/kg for the ketamine and 0.25 – 0.5 mg/kg for the xylazine and

finds there is no adverse effect on the heart. Anaesthesia lasts 4 – 15 minutes and the bird is perching in about 30 – 40 minutes.

There is some individual species response to this drug combination and Redig (1983) has worked out the optimum dose for a number of species of raptors. In general a sliding scale of doses which is approximately equivalent to 30 mg/kg of the ketamine for birds in the 100 – 150 gram range, 20 mg/kg for those near to 400 g in weight and 10 mg/kg for larger birds weighing one kilogram or slightly more. In eagles weighing 4 – 5 kg Redig uses 4.5 mg/kg. Haigh considers, and it is also the author's experience, that the nocturnal raptors metabolize the drugs more rapidly than diurnal raptors. The author has also recorded (Coles, 1984a) that the genus *Buteo* seems unusually sensitive to this drug combinination when used intramuscularly—going into deep anaesthesia, sometimes with apneoa—and that recovery times were prolonged. Redig (1983) also found that the Goshawk and Coopers Hawk needed higher doses and that recovery time was prolonged. Steiner & Davis gave 50 mg/kg of ketamine together with 10 mg/kg xylazine intramuscularly in the budgerigar. These workers consider that induction and recovery are somewhat rough.

The author has used this drug combination on a wide range of species and found it to be safe and effective. The dose used is 20 mg/kg of ketamine and 4 mg/kg of xylazine given intramuscularly. The bird is weighed and the dose of ketamine computed. An equal volume of xylazine is then added. Signs of sedation occur within a few minutes and induction is complete in 5 – 7 minutes. Using this dose anaesthesia lasts 10 – 20 minutes and birds are usually standing and able to perch in 1 – 2 hours. There is incoordination and sometimes a little excitement during recovery so that it is best to loosely roll the bird in a sheet of paper towel.

The combination is not satisfactory in the pigeons or doves and several authors, Forbes (1984), Green & Simpkin (1984), Samour (1984) and Coles (1984a), have all recorded that it is not satisfactory in the Galinules. Also *it is unsafe in the long-legged birds* which are liable to damage themselves during recovery. In penguins there is a prolonged recovery period.

General anaesthesia using volatile anaesthetics

Administration and anaesthetic circuits

Volatile anaesthetics can be given by using an open drop technique into the mouth or nares, by using an anaesthetic chamber or administered from an anaesthetic machine.

When using the open drop technique the only safe drug is methoxyflurane. It is dropped from a T.B. or 1 ml syringe into the mouth and given to effect.

A custom-made glass box is best used as an anaesthetic chamber for small birds. A piece of cotton wool is taped to the side of the container and a measured amount of the volatile anaesthetic allowed to soak into the cotton wool. Alternatively, the volatile anaesthetic in oxygen can be fed into the chamber via a small bore tube from the anaesthetic machine. The gas mixture may be delivered directly from an anaesthetic machine and into a mask. Whichever method is used for induction, the bird is maintained on the volatile anaesthetic preferably by connecting it to the anaesthetic machine using an endotracheal tube in all birds above about 300 g in body weight; in smaller birds a mask must be used. It is safer to use an Ayre's T-piece system since in only the very large birds is the tidal volume sufficient to move anaesthetic gas through a closed circuit. The author has used a Waters' to-and-fro system in the adult swan. The Rees' modification of the Ayre's T-piece, by using an open-ended rebreathing bag attached to the exhaust limb of the T-piece, is not necessary except in birds above 2 kg in weight. The most useful T-piece is the Bethune 'T' which has minimum dead space and can be connected to the 'Imp' respiratory monitor (see p. 108).

Endotracheal tubes

Plastic endotracheal tubes oral/nasal size 2.5 mm and 3.0 mm suitable for birds down to the size of a pigeon are manufactured by Portex*. Rubber, uncuffed endotracheal tubes sizes 3 or 4 can be used for slightly larger birds such as some Amazon parrots or macaws. A canine urinary catheter can be adapted by cutting the end obliquely and smoothing the end in a flame. The length of all tubes should be reduced as far as is practical to reduce the dead space. The tube should loosely fit in the glottis to allow the escape of gas around it so that there is no danger of over inflating the air sacs. If the bird is in light anaesthesia, particularly when using ketamine, there may be some temporary apnoea after the tube is passed. This can be overcome by using 1–2 drops of 2% lignocaine with adrenaline on the glottis.

* Portex Ltd., Kent, England.

Do not use a xylocane spray. The metered dose (10 mg) is toxic and there is no adrenaline to control absorption. The glottis can be seen just behind the root of the tongue. In some birds (e.g. cockerel and heron) the glottis is further back in the oropharynx and in the parrots the bulbous tongue hides the glottis. In all cases entubation of the trachea is made easier if the tongue is pulled forward. The tube should be lubricated and good spot lighting is advantageous.

The use of a mask may be the only practical way of maintaining small birds on volatile anaesthesia. Suitable masks can be made by cutting the base off a small plastic bottle (Fig. 5.2). The author has a selection of various sizes ready-made. Tall plastic bottles can be used to make masks for birds with long beaks (e.g sandpipers, herons and toucans). If the plastic is transparent then the eye can be seen during anaesthesia.

A number of gaseous anaesthetics have been successfully used in birds.

Ether

This agent is highly soluble in the plasma and therefore if it is used as the sole anaesthetic for both induction and maintainence, the initiation and recovery from anaesthesia is prolonged. The speed of induction and the rate of recovery from volatile anaesthetics is inversely proportional to the solubility of the anaesthetic in the plasma.

The use of ether is described by Sykes (1964) who administered it in air to chickens for up to 60 minutes. This worker noticed an initial drop in blood pressure when the ether is first given but this soon returns to normal. The author has used ether and had no problems but it has been superseded by better agents. Its main disadvantage is that it is highly inflammable and, as a T-piece system is being used, the room soon becomes filled with the pungent vapour.

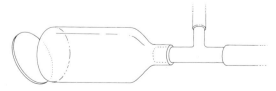

Fig. 5.2. Method of constructing a small anaesthetic face mask from a plastic bottle with the base removed.

Cyclopropane

Its use in chickens was first described by Hill & Noakes (1964). These workers used a 25 – 40% mixture in oxygen to maintain anaesthesia using a closed circuit system after induction with pentabarbitone. The anaesthesia was sometimes maintained for three hours. The anaesthesia produced was excellent and recovery was rapid. It is now rarely used because of its highly explosive potential—even to static electricity.

Halothane

This anaesthetic has been used by many people amongst whom are Marley & Payne (1964), Jones (1966), Graham-Jones (1966). The author has been using this agent on birds for the last 25 years, often as the sole anaesthetic. Many of these anaesthetic sessions have lasted over an hour and Marley & Payne used it for up to three hours. Jones (1977) considers that there is a great risk of overdosage. However, in the author's opinion, once the clinician understands the physiology of the avian respiratory system, and administers the drug accordingly, it is safe. Halothane is relatively insoluble in plasma so that induction and recovery of anaesthesia is rapid. Although some workers like to induce anaesthesia with 3 – 4% halothane in an oxygen flow of 0.5 – 2.0 litres, the author prefers to introduce the anaesthetic slowly, gradually increasing the concentration from 0.5 – 1% and raising this to 2.5 – 3% until the desired level of anaesthesia is reached. It is seldom necessary to go above 3%. Induction by this method takes longer but if the bird is struggling there is less chance of having the posterior air sacs filled with concentrated anaesthetic, should apnoea occur.

The practitioner should be aware that if an older type of Fluotec vapourizer is used, before the Mark III, much higher concentrations of anaesthetic are given if the flow rate is low.

Halothane can be given with 50% nitrous oxide and induction is somewhat smoother. It is unwise to increase the ratio of nitrous oxide above 50% because of the danger of hypoxia.

Birds can usually be maintained on 2.0 – 2.5% halothane if this is the sole anaesthetic agent. If an injectable drug has been used for induction then the bird can often be maintained at a lower level of 0.5 – 1.5%.

Redig (1983) considers the only disadvantage of halothane is that it requires an expensive precision vapouriser for its safe application. However the author has, and still sometimes administers it using a Boyle's type vapouriser, or trilene bottle.

Methoxyflurane

This anaesthetic is more soluble in plasma than halothane so that induction and recovery take longer. This agent has a wide margin of safety and is generally considered to be the safest of the volatile anaesthetics. However, Redig (1983) found it dangerous in *Bald Eagles,* which went into apnoea within one minute of its use and required mechanical ventilation.

Induction with methoxyflurane can be carried out using 3.5 – 4% and this takes approximately 8 – 10 minutes. The bird can then be maintained on 1.5 – 2.0%. This anaesthetic can be given without an expensive vapouriser but this is probably more wasteful. Because methoxyflurane has a high boiling point it is difficult to achieve a concentration above 3.5%. The anaesthetic is a good analgesic and analgesia apparently persists after recovery. The drug is absorbed into the fat depots from which it is gradually released and metabolised in the liver. Its main disadvantage is cost which at present is approximately four times that of halothane.

Anaesthetic emergencies

Apnoea

The most likely causes are too much anaesthetic, the toxicity of the anaesthetic and hypercapnoea. Apnoea will also occur after primary cardiac arrest.

Switch off any volatile anaesthetic and nitrous oxide. Increase the flow rate of oxygen and start mechanical ventilation immediately. This can be achieved by intermittently occluding the exhaust arm of the Ayer's T-piece with the finger. Quite satisfactory ventilation can be obtained in all but the larger birds by this method. In small birds even if an endotracheal tube is not in place, providing the oxygen flow rate is relatively high (e.g. 2 litres per minute), adequate ventilation can be carried out. Do not over-ventilate—the aim is to get a moderate excursion of the abdominal wall together with slight movement of the thorax. Over-ventilation washes out carbon dioxide and inhibits the chemoreceptors stimulating respiration. If very forceful, it may rupture the air sacs.

If a volatile anaesthetic is not in use it is still important to have an endotracheal tube in place so that artificial respiration can be carried out. Trying to ventilate a bird artificially by pressure on the sternum is not likely to be very effective and may cause damage to the ribs, liver or other organs.

If spontaneous respiration does not start within 2–3 minutes of artificial respiration give doxapram* at the rate of 7 mg/kg (0.3 ml/kg). This can be diluted 1:3 and given to a large bird by slow intravenous injection. In small- or medium- sized birds it can be dropped into the mouth so that it is absorbed through the mucous membrane.

Depression of the respiratory rate during a long period of anaesthesia

Stop the operative procedure. There may be a build up of $PaCO_2$. Increase the oxygen flow rate and gently artificially ventilate to wash out anaesthetic from the air sacs.

A blocked endotracheal tube

This may be indicated by more forceful and exaggerated respiratory movement. Clicking, gurgling or high-pitched squeaking sounds that could be mistaken for the bird awakening, all indicate some obstruction to the airway. Cyanosis is not usually seen except perhaps in chickens, and by the time this is recognized it usually too late to rectify the situation.

Remove the tube, blow it out, or preferably replace it with another tube. If there still appears to be some mucus present aspirate using a syringe and catheter.

Cardiac arrest

This usually occurs sometime after respiratory arrest. Marley & Payne (1964) using halothane anaesthesia in chickens noted there was a lag of about 10 minutes between respiratory and cardiac arrest. Unless some method of monitoring the heart is in use it will not be

* Dopram-V injection (A.H. Robins Co. Ltd.).

appreciated that cardiac arrest has actually occurred. The practitioner can try intermittent digital pressure on the sternum but this is not usually very successful, neither are intra-cardiac injections of adrenaline or lignocaine.

Suggested anaesthetic routines

(1) Short procedures lasting no more than 10 minutes where a quick recovery is required

There is little doubt that halothane administered in a gas flow of 50% oxygen and 50% nitrous oxide is the best anaesthetic for all species for quick procedures requiring general anaesthesia. However it *must* be administered *carefully* and slowly, preferably from an accurate vaporizer. Never increase the concentration to more than 3% and reduce this as soon as a satisfactory level of anaesthesia is reached.

Methoxyflurane is safe but is more expensive and induction and recovery take much longer. In large birds always consider whether local anaesthesia may be more applicable.

(2) For prolonged anaesthesia where this may be required for a period of up to an hour or more

The following routine is satisfactory for most species except those listed at the end of this section.

Anaesthesia is induced with a mixture of ketamine and xylazine given intramuscularly and the bird is maintained on 0.5–1.5% halothane given in 50% oxygen and 50% nitrous oxide.

If practical, weigh the bird and compute the dose of ketamine at 20 mg/kg. An equal volume of xylazine is added (giving 4 mg/kg). If it is not practical to weigh the bird, estimate its weight from the tables given at the back of this book. Give 75% of the computed dose intramuscularly. Wait five minutes, if narcosis is sufficient proceed with the volatile anaesthetic. If the bird is not sufficiently sedated give a further 50% the computed dose (i.e. at 20 mg/kg). Wait a further five minutes before giving any gaseous anaesthetic.

Always use an endotracheal tube wherever possible.

The use of atropine at the rate of 0.05–0.1 mg/kg (0.1–0.6 ml/kg of 600 mcg/ml solution) given at the same time as the ketamine and xylazine increases the safety margin of this technique.

When using this routine on raptors take particular care with the genus *Buteo*. In this group of birds it is wiser to start with a lower initial dose of 10 mg/kg of the ketamine. Also note the differential scale of doses mentioned earlier in the chapter (p. 114).

This anaesthetic technique is not suitable for galinules, pigeons, turacoes, hornbills, vultures or long-legged birds.

(a) Intravenous alphaxalone-alphadolone

This is the most suitable technique for the above-mentioned group of birds. In the smaller specimens the drug may be given intramuscularly but the results are not so consistent. Weigh the bird wherever possible. Use 10 mg/kg in birds below 1 kg and 4–5 mg/kg intravenously for birds over 3 kg and 36 mg/kg intramuscularly. Premedication with atropine probably increases the safety margin. Once respirations and heart rate are regular, slowly introduce the volatile anaesthetic (halothane) to maintain the anaesthesia.

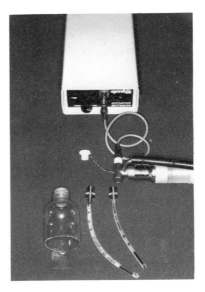

Fig. 5.3 The Imp respiratory monitor, which can be used with all species of birds to weight above 100 g.

6 / Surgery

General Considerations

Selection of avian patients for surgery

Before carrying out any sort of operation on a bird it is wise to carry out a thorough clinical examination. Obviously, birds which are in a state of shock due to trauma are bad surgical risks. The obese budgerigar which has been confined to its cage throughout life is also a bad risk. However, the author has been surprised on a number of occasions by birds which have been abnormally thin and in poor condition which have survived anaesthesia and surgery. If possible, it is better to try to improve the nutritional state of these patients first. Probably the bird at greatest risk is the one with an obvious respiratory problem. Any bird that is dyspnoeic or one that becomes dyspnoeic with the minimum of handling is a bad surgical risk. A bird that has ascites or a large abdominal space occupying mass is a bad risk.

Positioning of the patient during surgery

Any bird placed in dorsal recumbency will have a reduced air sac volume, so that in birds with space occupying lesions of the abdomen this condition is exacerbated. This problem is discussed in more detail in Chapter 5, p. 106. Although the vast majority of surgical patients can be placed on their backs and are less liable to be moved in this position, it is better to have them in ventral or lateral recumbency. When in lateral recumbency care should be taken not to forcibly fold the wings too far back above the body, as this may restrict respiratory movement.

Essential equipment

A selection of small instruments such as those used in ophthalmic or micro-surgery should be used. The following list is the most useful and the minimum that should be available.
(1)   4.5″ (114 mm) enucleation or strabismus scissors

(2) Tissue forceps with 1 × 2 teeth such as Lister's conjunctival forceps.

(3) Straight Halsted mosquito forceps

(4) Curved Halsted mosquito forceps

(5) A blunt-ended probe. Sterile cotton wool buds will serve this purpose and will also act as swabs for clearing blood or exudate.

(6) Fine needle holders

(7) A Spreull needle attached to a sterile 10 ml syringe is useful for suction or irrigation.

(8) Suitable suturing materials, e.g. No. 2 pseudo monofilament Polyamide,* 3/0 Chromic cat gut or Polyglactin[†] 910 swaged onto round-bodied, taper-cut pointed needles. If absorbable sutures are used in the skin the bird will not need handling again for suture removal.

When using instruments for delicate surgery the hands are under better control if the surgeon is seated and it may be possible to rest the elbows on the table. Also some form of magnification combined with good illumination is advisable. An operating microscope is the ultimate choice but this is costly. Binocular loupes or magnifying spectacles are also useful. The least expensive system is a combined lens and circular fluorescent light. This is marketed by several surgical instrument companies and a number of different designs are used in industry by persons carrying out delicate work. Harrison (1984) suggests mounting the fibre optic laparoscope (see Chapter 2) on a flexible arm, like that used for some table lamps, and using this for magnification and lighting. This gives excellent lighting and magnification but the field of vision is somewhat restricted.

Haemorrhage

There is little doubt that many avian surgical patients die of blood loss. Systemic blood pressures in birds are high compared to mammals. Blood loss from severed vessels is therefore rapid and the control of bleeding is of paramount importance, particularly in small birds. However, Kovách *et al.* (1968 and 1969) have demonstrated that several species of birds are able to tolerate blood loss better than

---

* 'Supramid' (Armour Pharmaceutical Co. Ltd.).
[†] 'Vicryl' (Ethicon Ltd.).

mammals. Circulating blood volume is usually little more than 10% of body weight (see p. 20), yet Kovách has shown that pigeons can survive blood loss of 8% of body weight during prolonged haemorrhage. Although the blood pressure and heart rate dropped these returned to normal within one half to four hours. This effect is apparently due to the greatly increased capillary surface area (3–5 times that found in the domestic cat) that is available for the absorbtion of reserve tissue fluid and to a very pronounced vasoconstriction in the skeletal muscles. From the practical point of view the author has often noticed that birds presented at the surgery because of trauma have suffered considerable blood loss, as shown by their surroundings, and yet they have survived.

The arterial capillaries in the muscles are more influenced by autonomic nervous control than by the level of local metabolites (H^+, CO_2 and lactic acid) than is the case in mammals. Consequently premedication with atropine prior to surgery may help to control haemorrhage. Although the resting heart rate of many birds is lower than that in mammals of comparable size, stress or excitement very soon leads to a much more rapid heart rate. Struggling due to an inadequate depth of anaesthesia can result in considerable haemorrhage. Harrison (1984) has used blood transfusions in birds. It has been shown that blood from heterogenous species can safely be used for a first transfusion (p. 104). However, blood for transfusion is unlikely to be readily available and in view of the above mentioned observations of Kovách et al. the discrete use of blood volume expanders such as Haemace 1* is all that is necessary.

Cleaning and antisepsis of the operation site

To obtain a clear operating area every feather has to be meticulously plucked. If cut, the feather does not grow until the bird's next moult. Plucking can be tedious and it sometimes is easier using forceps. The shaft of the feather must be firmly gripped and pulled out cleanly so that the germinal layer of the feather papilla is not damaged and the feather will regenerate. Regeneration will occur in most cases within a few weeks of plucking. If the feather is fully grown, it is a dead structure which will not bleed when plucked. If the feather is plucked before growth is completed and the feather has not completely

* 'Haemacel' (Behring inst.).

Only the minimum number of feathers consistent with clearing the
operation site should be plucked to avoid excessive heat loss,
particularly in small birds. For the same reason the surgical site
should be cleansed with minimal antiseptic solution. Cleaning and
sterilization can be carried out using a quaternary ammonium
solution* Chlorhexidine‡, Benzalkonium Chloride§ or one of the
tamed iodine antiseptics such as Povidone¶ iodine.

To limit heat loss the patient should be placed on an electrically
heated pad or on a rigid hot water bottle covered in sterile cloths.

Surgery of the skin and associated structures

Overall the skin of birds is much thinner than that of mammals of
comparable size. In the feathered areas the thickness and strength
varies between the feather tracts (pterylae) and the featherless areas
between these tracts (apteria). In the apteria the dermis has a stronger
mesh of collagen fibres (Stettenheim 1972).

Surgical incisions are best made in the apteria, parallel and mid-way
between the adjacent feather tracts, and the subsequent sutures
placed in the apteria.

The subcutis and dermis contain only a few horizontal sheets of
elastic fibres so that avian skin is not very elastic. The skin is not firmly
attached to the underlying muscle, but in some areas (the skull, the
carpus, the digits, the pelvis) the skin is firmly and extensively
attached to bone. Avian skin is therefore not very mobile and easily
tears, particularly where it attached to bone. The skin is best sutured
using suture material swaged on to atraumatic needles. There are
numerous blood vessels, both capillary and larger vessels, within the
skin and haemorrhage can be a problem. When possible, incisions
should be made with an electro-surgical or ophthalmic diathermy
knife. The scalpel should not be used at all for most types of avian
surgery. If diathermy or ophthalmic cautery is not available an
incision can be made by nicking and blunt dissection with scissors.

Lacerated wounds

These are sometimes caused by attacks from aviary mates or flying into sharp objects, particularly during stormy and gusty weather. Racing pigeons not uncommonly return home having been blown into telephone or barbed wire. If these wounds involve the anterior sternum, as they often do, there may be damage to the clavicular air sac with resulting subcutaneous emphysema. This usually resolves spontaneously, but if necessary, can be deflated with a hypodermic needle and syringe. Providing the wound is fresh and haemorrhage has been controlled the wound can be treated on a routine basis and usually heals by first intention without secondary infection.

Subcutaneous abscesses

These are not uncommon around the head, particularly in parrots. They often involve the paranasal sinuses around the eye but also occur in the submandibular region. These abscesses are usually filled with inspissated, caseous pus. The abscess should be opened with a scalpel fitted with a No. 11 blade, by inserting the point first and directing the cutting edge away from the bird. The pus is then scooped out and the cavity curetted. A Volkmann's spoon can be used, but a useful instrument for a small bird is a canine tooth scaler with a rounded spatulate end. When opening a submandibular abscess care should be taken to avoid the large subcutaneous blood vessels in this region. Before suturing the skin, a bacteriological swab should be taken for culture and antibiotic-sensitivity testing. An injection of ampicillin may be given at the time of opening the abscess although this antibiotic may need to be changed later in the light of the results of bacteriological culture. In the case of very small birds of 15–20 g size it may not be practical to suture an abscess after opening. In this case the cavity can be cauterized with a silver nitrate pencil and left to heal by granulation.

   Abscesses sometimes occur around and in the ear. The surrounding skin can become thickened and the ear canal filled with exudate. These abscesses need great care because of the risk of haemorrhage and damage to the tympanum which is relatively near the surface. It may be wiser to try and first reduce the swelling with topical steroids combined with antibiotics.

Feather cysts

These are usually seen in the region of the carpus but can occur in other parts of the body. The author has never seen them in the many thousands of wild birds he has examined. They are most often seen in some breeds of canary but do occur in other captive birds. They may be genetic in origin or caused by mechanical damage to the developing feather follicle or excessive preening by the bird. They are usually dry and contain the remains of the undeveloped feather which has been unable to emerge in a normal manner from the follicle. However, some neoplasms may look like feather follicles and bleed profusely when opened. Since the feather follicle persists in maintaining an abnormal direction these cysts will recur if they are merely opened. The whole section of skin including the cyst should be carefully dissected out. Dissection is not easy without damaging the neighbouring follicles and the skin is adherent to the underlying bone in this area.

Subcutaneous tumours and cysts

These are seen in all species but are most common in the psittacine birds, particularly the budgerigar. They are not usually invasive but can become ulcerated. They are usually easily dissected free of surrounding tissue by using a closed pair of mosquito haemostats. Great care should be taken to search out and clamp any blood vessels supplying the neoplasm. This is particularly the case with the common lipomatous tumours found over the thorax of the budgerigar which often have a large blood vessel beneath them and which can bleed profusely. Meticulous attention should be given to any haemorrhage into the wound post operatively. For this reason any loose skin left after removing a large tumour should be trimmed and dead space diminished.

Fatty tumours in budgerigars are best reduced prior to surgery by strict dietary and medical routines. This also improves the general physical condition of the bird. The seed should be rationed to one heaped teaspoonful twice daily. Add soluble vitamins and diluted Lugol's iodine to the drinking water.

Tumours of the uropygial or preen gland

These may be benign adenomas or malignant adenocarcinomas that can become adherent to the underlying bone. Haemorrhage is not usually a problem but if the tumour has been allowed to reach an appreciable size some difficulty may be experienced in repair. Removal of the preen gland does not seem to have any adverse effects.

It does not seem essential to the maintenance of budgerigar plumage and it may not be essential to other species of birds since it is absent in some species such as many pigeons, parrots, emus, cassowaries and bustards (King & McLelland, 1975b). The composition of the secretion varies in different species but usually contains a complex of water repellent waxes, lipids and proteins. It may also contain a precursor of vitamin D (Stettenheim, 1972). The vitamin D precursor may only be important in growing birds.

The head region

Accidental wounds

Apart from fractures of the beak, dealt with below, other fractures are liable to result in instant death. However, less serious injury may cause damage to the skin including the eyelids. The skin over the whole of the skull in most species is not very elastic and is adherent to the bone. Any wound more than a few days old will have contracted with resultant fibrosis and it will be difficult to suture the skin edges together. If the upper eyelid is damaged at the nasal canthus it may be possible to slide the remaining part of the eyelid forward, by making a lateral canthotomy, as shown in Fig. 6.1. Do not remove a wedge of skin below this incision, as is sometimes done in the mammals for this type of plastic surgery. In the bird this only results in too much tension across the lower eyelid. In birds it is the lower eyelid that carries out most of the movement in covering the eyeball.

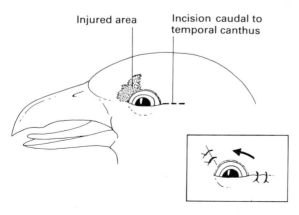

Fig. 6.1. Position of incisions for suturing damage to upper lid.

Enucleation of the eye

Before this is undertaken the following factors should be taken into account. The eye in birds is relatively much larger than in mammals of comparable size, particularly in raptors. In fact, avian eyes are much larger than they appear to the casual observer and occupy more space in the skull than the brain. The extra occular muscles have been greatly reduced in size and the resulting loss of movement in the eyeball is compensated for by an increased movement of the whole head supported by the very flexible neck. Reduction in the eye muscles has resulted in much less space for the surgeon to work between the eyeball and its socket. The globe of the eyeball is much more rigid than in the mammal. Not only is the sclera cartilagenous but there is a ring of bony plates around the circumference near the corneal scleral junction. There is only a thin interorbital septum between the two eyes, which is particularly evident in the owls. In removing one eye the optic nerve of the other eye can easily be damaged. At the back of the eye in some species there is a U-shaped bone in the sclera surrounding the optic nerve. There is a well developed venous plexus near the cornea-scleral junction.

The simplest method of enucleation is by lateral canthotomy, then an incision of the cornea to remove the aqueous, the lens and the vitreous. The sclera and choroid should then be carefully collapsed into the resulting free space using scissors and forceps. It may be wiser to leave the back of the sclera with the attached tissues intact and to plug the socket with an absorbent fibrin or gelatin sponge. The eyelids are then sutured together after removing the margin of each lid.

Tumours of the nictitating membrane are occasionally seen in birds. Apart from the cosmetic aspect, which worries the owner, the surgeon should always consider whether the removal of this membrane is absolutely necessary. As in mammals, but probably more so in birds, the nictitating membrane has a very important protective function to the eye. Removal of the membrane can lead to a keratitis.

Cannulation of the infra-orbital sinuses

This is a simple procedure that can be carried out in a quiet bird without anaesthetic. It may be required in any species with a chronic sinusitis (see section on clinical examination of the head) the point of entry is illustrated in Fig. 6.2. In bad cases the sinus is well-distended

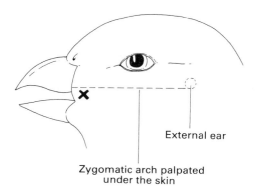

External ear

Zygomatic arch palpated
under the skin

Fig. 6.2. The X-cross shows the point of entry for cannulation of the infra-orbital sinuses.

and entry can be made without any difficulty into the area of greatest distension. In the budgerigar the hypodermic needle needs only to be advanced horizontally to a depth of approximately 2 mm. A suitable volume of fluid for injection is 0.1–0.3 ml. Excess fluid will exit through the nares and may also flow into the pharynx so care must be taken that none flows down the glottis.

Hyperkeratinization of the cere and nares

In budgerigars a horn-like projection sometimes develops from the cere and occasionally may obstruct the nares (see Fig. 1.2). This is purely excessive keratin that has not desquamated from the basal tissues. It is dry and bloodless and can be cut with scissors or nail clippers, care being taken not to go too close to the sensitive cere.

The larger psittacines may also develop rhinolyths or collections of dry exudate within the nares which can act like a ball valve. They may partially obstruct breathing and cause annoyance. It is a simple matter to scoop these out with a dental scaler.

Abscesses in the oral cavity

These can occur anywhere in the mouth. They may be seen around and partly blocking the choanal opening from the nasal cavity or on the tongue, particularly in parrots. They should be opened and thoroughly curretted. It is not practical to suture those over the choanal opening so they should be cauterized.

Beak problems

Deformities and overgrowth

Budgerigars often are seen with overgrown or distorted beaks. There is very little than can be done surgically to correct these defects. Regular clipping with nail clippers is the best routine. Other psittacines also get overgrown beaks sometimes through lack of proper wear or they may become distorted through excessive wear caused by climbing the metal bars of their cage. Metabolic bone disease not only affects the other parts of the skeleton but also affects growth of the premaxilla and mandible so that the overlying beak becomes distorted. The rhamphotheca or heavily cornified covering of the beak is a constantly growing structure. The cornified surface of the tissue obliquely slides towards the tip of the beak (Stettenheim, 1972), the edges and surface of which are continually worn away during use. Falconers regularly 'cope' or cut the upper beaks of their birds to counteract overgrowth.

In all cases the beak can be trimmed to shape (not just cut off square) with nail clippers and then smoothed off with fine sandpaper. An emery board is very suitable. If bleeding occurs, it can be cauterized with a silver nitrate pencil or solution of ferric chloride after which it is neutralized with sodium chloride. Occasionally a beak is seen that has either developed abnormally from hatching or has been fractured and allowed to heal in an uncorrected position. The lower beak may stick out at an angle to the upper beak. The owner might think this is due to dislocation, but because of the double articulation of the avian lower jaw (Fig. 6.3), dislocation is unlikely. There are two joints of the quadrate bone, dorsally with the temporal bone and ventrally with the articular bone, that distribute any disrupting force applied to the mandible.

There may be prehension difficulty with soft food tending to lodge at the side of the beak. There are two methods of dealing with this problem—both of which require osteotomy. Firstly, the difference in the lengths of the two sides is measured carefully. Procedure number one is to remove a section of bone from the longer of the two mandibles and then wire the bone back in position with one or two stainless steel wire sutures. The second technique is to use a sliding osteotomy. This is carried out just anterior to the commissure of the integument covering the upper and lower beaks. In this area the bone is fairly accessible and there are no large blood vessels overlying the

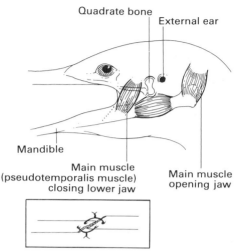

Fig. 6.3. Diagrammatic representation of the articulation of the mandible in a typical bird, showing one method of osteotomy. The dotted line indicates where the bone is sectioned.

bone. The pseudotemporalis muscle closing the beak overlies the posterior part of the section to be made in the bone. The size of this muscle depends on the species and the power of closing the beak, which depends on the bird's feeding habits. Fortunately, most of those birds where the operation is required have weak pseudotemporalis muscles and relatively long, straight mandibles. The part of the muscle which may overlie that part of the bone to be sectioned is partly freed from its insertion onto the bone. Having decided on the direction of the oblique section through the bone a line of fine holes is drilled along this position. The bone then cut with a saw. The anterior part of the mandible can then be slid cranially in relation to its posterior half and again wired in position with stainless steel wire sutures. If the upper pair of holes drilled for the wire are large enough, they will take a catgut, or better, polyglactin* suture as well as the stainless steel suture. This absorbable suture can be used to hold the pseudotemporalis muscle back in place (Fig. 6.3).

   In carrying out both these methods, the integument covering the bone needs to be carefully stripped for a little way down on each side of the section through the bone. As far as is practical it is better to try and suture the integument so that the suture line does not lie over the

* 'Vicryl' (Ethicon Ltd.).

union in the bone but more to one side. For sectioning the bone a sterile junior hacksaw blade can be used. This is sometimes easier if the blade is first snapped in half. The wire sutures should be tight enough only to bring the bone together, overtightening usually results in the wire cutting its way through the fine trabecula structure of the bone. Birds show little discomfort after both these procedures and are surprisingly rough with their beaks. They usually start to feed straight away. Because of this some external support is recommended. Often an aluminium finger splint can be cut down and bent into shape to form a sort of cradle to the mandible. This can then be wired into position with the wire going through the skin and over the bone. The success of these operations will depend not only on the skill of the surgeon but also on the right selection of cases. The temperament of the bird is important. Ducks usually make good subjects. Success also depends on the size and shape of the lower beak. One needs a relatively long and straight area on which to operate. One disadvantage of these operations is that the mandiblular branch of the 5th cranial nerve runs through a canal in the mandible and is quite likely to be destroyed when the bone is sectioned. When using the second method in a reasonably large bird it may be possible to cut carefully round the circumference of the bone providing the predrilling has not already damaged the nerve. However, the nerve distal to this area is only sensory and the bird is not apparently affected by anaesthesia of this area.

Splits or fractures

If the damage is a simple crack in the bone, particularly if only one side is affected, then a stainless steel wire suture will suffice. If only the cornified integument is damaged it can often simply be glued back in position using an epoxy resin glue or one of the 'super glues'.

If the beak is more seriously damaged and is hanging by the intact integument, something more robust than simple wire suturing will be needed. Various methods have been used by different workers. These methods nearly always involve the use of Steinmann's pins or Kirschner wires placed in a cruciate pattern. These are further braced with figures-of-eight stainless wire sutures placed around the ends of the pins. The ends of the pins are best protected by an epoxy resin glue or similar substance. Some sort of cradling device as described above, to give external support is advised.

Partial loss of the beak

This can happen in any species but is commonest in those birds with rather large or long beaks such as the hornbill, the toucan, parrots, ducks and, occasionally, wading birds. In this last group, because of the long, thin beak, the problem is insoluble. In those birds with a wider base to the beak it may be possible to fit a prosthesis. If only the tip of the beak is broken off, particularly if this does not involve the underlying premaxillae, the beak can be filed and shaped with sandpaper. Eventually the beak will return to normal.

If a small part of the premaxilla is missing, the open end needs to be first plugged before shaping. A surgical glue such as a self-curing acrylic is preferable but if this is not available epoxy resin glues* such as those used for car body repair kits can be used and do not appear toxic when used externally.

There are few papers in the scientific literature that record the fitting of a prosthesis. Von Becker (1974) reports a problem in two hornbill ravens, damaged in transit, that was repaired by fitting steel plating to cover the ends of the remaining stumps. Most other reports have used a beak moulded from fibreglass or dental acrylic. The material marketed under the name of 'Technovit 609'† is suitable. The author on two occasions has used high density polyethylene for a prosthesis fitted to two parrots and has used polypropamide to replace a duck's partly-missing upper beak. In the last case the polypropamide upper beak was fashioned from the barrel of a 10 ml plastic syringe. Approximately one-third of the circumference of the plastic tube was used and was found to have about the right curvature. This was then overlapped on the remaining proximal half of the beak and kept in position with stainless steel wire sutures. The bird started to feed as soon as it recovered from the anaesthetic.

In the parrot cases the prostheses were carved from a block of high-density polyethylene, the material used for making human artificial hips. The problem in both cases is the satisfactory and permanent fixation of the prosthesis to the remainder of the beak. A surgical glue can be used, or wire sutures or Kirschner wires used in a cruciate pattern. In all cases the attachment eventually works loose due to the birds' constant rough usage and to pressure erosion of the

* 'Araldyte' (Ciba-Geigy); 'Plastic Padding' (Aktie bolaget).
† (Kulzer & Co. GmbH.).

bone. The bone, in any case, is not very solid in the region of the nares, being composed of a mesh of interlocking trabeculae enclosed in a thin, outer shell. Nature has provided a very strong and light-weight structure admirably adapted to the function of prehension for the particular species but quite useless as a firm anchorage in orthopaedic surgery. The parrots used the prosthesis quite readily to climb both vertically and across the top of the cage. They did not use the beak to crack nuts. This may have been due to the fact that the natural beak has a number of transverse ridges across the internal surface. They are used in lodging a nut with the tongue in order to crack it with the force of the lower beak. The bird has to be maintained on soft foods such as seed, ground down in a food blender and mixed with peanut butter or mashed potato. These birds readily eat a variety of fruit. Oesophagotomy tubes may be required immediately post-operatively in some cases.

It is questionable whether the use of a prosthesis is always justified in parrots. Although the device is well tolerated, apart from the improved cosmetic effect, there may be little advantage to the bird. The birds soon learn to climb and to feed quite effectively on soft foods without an upper beak and appear to be quite happy once the original lesion has healed.

Surgery of the neck

Sometimes a foreign body will lodge in the oesophagus. This could be a long bone from the prey of a raptor or a fish hook in a water bird. The oesophagus in birds is wide and easily dilated, but the muscular wall is thin. It may be possible to extract the object via the oropharynx in the anaesthetised subject. In other cases an incision will have to be made in the neck. There are no particular problems but it is as well to make the incision on the left side since the jugular vein is better developed on the right side. The external carotid artery does not form until near the base of the skull and the internal carotids are tucked under the cervical vertebrae.

Impaction of the crop can occur. This can be felt as a plastic mass situated at the thoracic inlet. Providing an incision is made over the area of greatest distension there is little danger of damage to other structures. This is a simple operation and may be done under local anaesthesia. Both crop and skin should be sutured separately.

Devoicing birds

This is usually carried out on the domestic cockerel or a peacock. It is also recorded as having been performed on some raptors. It is questionable whether this is an ethical procedure for a veterinarian to perform in the light of the opinion on animal welfare in the United Kingdom. Some might consider this an unjustifiable mutilation. However, the technique is described for reference purposes.

The anaesthetized bird is placed on its back and positioned with the neck hanging over the edge of the table or over a sandbag to fully extend the ventral surface of the neck. A mid-line incision is made anterior to the sternum and well above the base of the neck. After reflecting the skin, the underlying muscle and fascia are carefully split to expose the thin-walled crop. This is separated and deflected to one side. The trachea and thoracic inlet are exposed and the trachea very carefully freed from surrounding structures. The syrinx lies well within the thoracic inlet under the sternum and the prominent

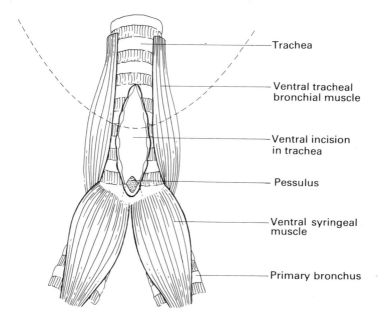

Fig. 6.4. The trachea, syrinx and main muscles of a typical bird, to show the position of the pessulus. The dotted line shows the level of the clavicles and thoracic inlet.

pectoral muscles. Very gentle traction on the trachea will bring it into view. The attachment of the trachea in the region of the syrinx is very delicate and easily torn. There is a network of small blood vessels around the syrinx (see Fig. 3.1) and these will have to be ligated at both ends. An incision is next made into the ventral surface of the trachea using small, sharp scissors. This incision extends as far as the pessulus or prismatic bone (Fig. 6.4). Using a small retractor or speculum to keep the trachea open a small electric cautery point is used to cauterize the anterior surface of the pessulus. The temperature of the cautery point should be tested before insertion and the electrical current should not be switched on until the instrument has been inserted and is touching the pessulus. After cautery the current should be switched off before the cautery point is removed. In this way it is less liable to stick in the tissues and cause haemorrhage through tearing. There is no need to suture the tracheal incision, the trachea should reform in shape. Muscle and skin are sutured. This method is that described by Durant (1953).

Another technique described to the author by Jordan (F.T.W., 1982; personal communication) is to incise the syringeal membranes, then to scarify the outside of the syrinx. A piece of stainless steel mesh is then wrapped around the syrinx so that the scarified area will adhere to this.

Abdominal surgery

The clinical indications for entering the avian abdomen are: (1) diagnostic, (2) the removal of foreign bodies from the proventriculus or gizzard, (3) the relief of an impacted gizzard or ventriculus, (4) the removal of tumours and (5) the relief of an impacted oviduct.

The approach to the abdomen is usually through a mid-line ventral incision but if a neoplasm of the gonads or adrenal gland is definitely diagnosed, a flank incision gives better access to these organs and their associated blood supply. The ventral incision is best made slightly to the (surgeon's) left of the mid-line.

The abdominal muscles are the same as those in the mammal but the extent of the linea alba and the thickness of the muscles varies according to the species of bird. It is best developed in strong flying birds. Harrison (1984) suggests extending the mid-line incision by incisions at right angles, parallel to the posterior edge of the sternum, so as to form two flaps. This produces better exposure but if these parasternal incisions are extended more than a third of the distance from the mid-line to the ribs in some species, the intestinal peritoneal cavity will be entered, which may not be necessary. Just below these outer areas lie the left and right posterior thoracic air sacs. Also depending on the species, the mid-line incision, if extended too far posteriorly, will enter the intestinal peritoneal cavity. This cavity contains the two abdominal air sacs. Taking the above anatomical facts into consideration it is not desirable to incise and deflate all four posterior air sacs (see Fig. 6.5).

If a careful incision is made through the linea alba, with blunt-pointed scissors, while picking it up with rat-toothed forceps to hold it away from the underlying viscera, entry is made into the right ventral hepatic cavity. On the floor of this cavity (anatomically the dorsal aspect of the cavity) is a membrane (right post hepatic septum) that resembles an air sac but is one of the peritoneal membranes. Contained within this first cavity, are the organs shown in Fig 6.6.

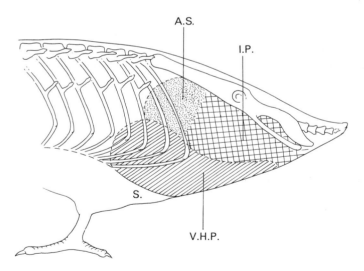

Fig. 6.5. Diagram showing the relative positions of the coelomic cavities. A.S., left and right caudal thoracic air sacs; I.P., left and right intestinal peritoneal cavities. The two cavities are divided by the dorsal mesentery in which is suspended the intestine and reproductive tract. Intimately connected with the intestine are the left and right abdominal air sacs; V.H.P., left and right ventral hepatic cavities. These are divided by the ventral mesentery. The cavities only contain the two lobes of the liver; S., sternum. After Dunker (1978).

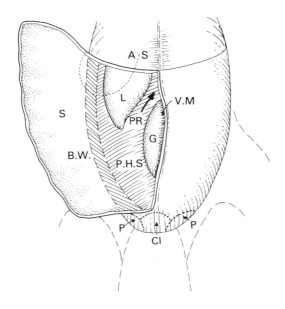

Fig. 6.6. Incision through the linea alba into the right ventral hepatic cavity. A.S., Dotted line shows the position of the right caudal thoracic air sac below the level of the ventral hepatic cavity containing the liver; L., right lobe of liver; P.R., the approach to the proventriculus; G., gizzard attached to linea alba by the ventral mesentery; P.H.S. right post hepatic septum distal to which lies the duodenum and pancreas in the intestinal peritoneal cavity and which is surrounded by the abdominal air sac; C.L., cloaca. An incision in this area will enter the intestinal peritoneal cavity; P., pubis; B.W., body wall; S., skin flap; V.M., ventral mesentery.

The gizzard is attached by the ventral mesentery to the abdominal wall at the mid-line. Distal to the ventral mesentery lies the left ventral hepatic cavity containing the left lobe of the liver. The ventral hepatic cavities contain no air sacs. The thickness and translucency of the post hepatic septal membranes vary with the size of the bird, (also if there is any degree of airsacculitis or peritonitis causing adhesions). In small birds the post hepatic septum acts as a fat depot, obscuring the intestine beneath. The air sacs are mostly adherent and supported by the surrounding tissues and so will not collapse if punctured. Providing entry into and destruction of the integrity of the air sacs is not extensive, it has no more effect on the respiratory system than tracheotomy does in mammals.

Gastrotomy

The muscular stomach or ventriculus is easily accessible through the initial abdominal incision. Its muscular wall varies in thickness; in the gizzard of some graniferous birds is very thick. In these species haemorrhage from the muscle can be a problem if a diathermy knife is not used.

The glandular part of the stomach or proventriculus is not quite so accessible but gentle traction on the ventriculus will bring the posterior part of this organ into view.

Surgical access to the rest of the alimentary canal

If it is necessary, an approach can be made via the route used by Durant (1926 and 1930) and Schlotthauer, *et al.* (1933) for ablation of the caecea. This is to make an incision medial and parallel to the left pubis. There is a large artery in this area that must be avoided. This approach gives access not only to the caecea but also to the rectum and the distal part of the ileum.

The duodenum and pancreas are best approached via a ventral abdominal incision. This is made through the mid-line into the right ventral hepatic cavity and then through the right post hepatic septum (described above), on the floor of this coelomic cavity, when the duodenum is found directly underneath. This surgical approach also gives access to the supraduodenal loop of the ileum and some other parts of the small intestine. However, the intestine in birds is not as mobile as in mammals, being not only suspended in the mesentery attached both dorsally and ventrally, but this mesentery is intimately surrounded by the abdominal air sacs. Any traction on the intestine is liable to lead to a tearing of these membranes and possible rupture of the associated blood vessels together with traction on and stimulation of the nerve of Remak containing the autonomic nerves.

The reproductive tract

Egg retention and egg peritonitis

Any lesion causing enlargement of the reproductive tract is likely to displace the stomach towards the right. An incision in the mid-line is therefore quite likely to pierce the ventral mesentery, by which the ventriculus is attached to the ventral abdominal wall, and to enter the left ventral hepatic cavity. On the floor of this and probably displaced upwards by the enlarged oviduct, will be the left post hepatic septum. Incision of this will expose the oviduct. If an egg is to be removed by hysterotomy it is best to put in one or two preplaced sutures before making the incision in the oviduct. Once this is opened the wall of the oviduct contracts and, being very thin, is difficult to suture.

If there is any fluid in the abdomen, as in egg peritonitis, Harrison (1984) suggests draining with a Penrose drain and flushing with antibiotics. This is carried out 2–3 days prior to hysterotomy in the case of an egg impacted in the oviduct. Instead of carrying out a laparotomy, Rosskopf & Woerpel, (1982) describe paracentesis of the egg contents by using a hypodermic needle pushed through the abdominal wall. When yolk and albumen have been extracted, the egg shell collapses and the bird is given an injection of oxytocin and calcium. The remains of the egg are then expelled within 2 days.

If part of the impacted egg can be seen through the cloacal opening, the needle can be inserted into the egg through this exposed section of shell.

An impacted egg sometimes leads to prolapse of the oviduct through the cloaca. If this is not dealt with quickly the tissues become congested, they can dry and eventually become necrotic. It is essential to moisten the prolapsed parts with normal saline. Use a lubricant such as petroleum jelly or liquid paraffin to ease the egg out through the opening in the prolapsed oviduct. The blunt end of a sterile thermometer is very useful for this purpose, being slowly rotated around the circumference between the egg and the wall of the oviduct.

After the egg has been removed the cloaca may remain prolapsed. This may also occur after normal egg laying in a weakened oviduct. Rosskopf, Woerpel & Pitts, (1983) described the use of No. 0 stainless steel wire sutures around the vent to retain the cloaca in a greater Sulfur-crested Cockatoo. These authors also describe cloacoplexy by suturing the abdominal wall to the cloaca. The cloaca is readily accessible through a mid-line incision between the 2 public bones. It should be noted that there is a danger that the prolapse may contain intestine, oviduct, or ureter and may lead to obstruction of these organs.

Neoplasia

Access to the ovary or adrenal gland, necessary because of a neoplasm may be made via a flank incision. Aranez & Sanguin (1955) give an excellent description of this approach for poulardization (removal of the ovary) in the domestic fowl. The incision is made over the last two left hand ribs (6th and 7th). The skin is first incised, the sartorius muscle is pushed posteriorly and the incision deepened between the two ribs. The aim is to keep close to the anterior border of the 7th rib to avoid the intercostal artery. The ribs are kept apart with a retractor. Below the ribs the left abdominal air sac is penetrated revealing the intestines which are pushed aside with a blunt probe. The ovary and adrenal gland should then be visible. In the normal immature organ the base can then be grasped with forceps and twisted off. The same technique can be applied to the testes.

In a bird smaller than the domestic fowl or one where the gonad is enlarged and neoplastic the situation can be more diffiuclt. The initial incision can be enlarged by removing the last two ribs. The blood vessels supplying the gonads are short and not extensible, unlike the case in the dog or cat. They are close to the dorsal aorta and vena cava, which can easily be damaged. Very good illumination, magnification and meticulous surgical technique is required for success. In many of these cases the approach made by Durant (1926 and 1930) and Schlotthauer et al. (1933) for ablation of the caecea as described above may give more operating room.

The penis

An occasional problem seen in male ducks is prolapse of the enlarged penis. This can be two or three inches long and drags on the ground. It can become dry and excoriated and necrotic. The cause is usually due to injury brought about by bullying from another drake. In the duck the penis is an extension of the mucous membrane lining the cloaca. There is no vascular corpus spongiosum as in the mammal. The only solution to the problem is amputation which seems to have little deleterious clinical effect except to make the duck ineffective for breeding purposes.

Repair of the ruptured abdominal wall

This is a difficult problem which is more common in the obese female budgerigar. The muscle is weakened by egg laying and infiltration of fat. Gradually the whole abdominal musculature is stretched apart along the line of the linea alba. The weight of the abdominal viscera causes marked enlargement and descent of all the structures so that the swelling becomes pendulant. The results are potentially serious with impaired respiratory and cardiac function. The liver may be enlarged and infiltrated with fat. These cases are bad surgical risks.

If successful anaesthesia can be achieved, with the bird in dorsal recumbency, it is best not to incise the body wall. This should be picked up so that the underlying viscera falls away, then alternative mattress sutures of 3/0 chromic catgut and non-absorbable 'Supramid'* are placed through skin and the muscle remaining at the edges of the hernia. The object is not to pull the body wall too tightly together but for the catgut to induce some fibrosis. It is hoped this will produce a renewed and stronger linea alba. Providing the suture needle is placed just below the skin it will not damage the underlying viscera, which are protected by the fat.

Orthopaedic surgery

Before attempting any surgery on the bones of birds it is well to take into account some general considerations. During evolution the avian skeleton has undergone structural responses to the engineering problems of support and movement imposed on a flying vertebrate. Although the elemental structure of the bone, which is a lattice of hydroxyapatite crystals intimately associated with a mesh of collagen fibrils, is basically the same as in mammals, the gross anatomy of the bone has changed. The bulk of an avian long bone is concentrated in a thin porcelain like shell which shows little or no organization into Haversian systems. The interior of the bone contains a network of struts or trabeculae, each one of which is orientated to counteract the external forces imposed on the bone at that particular point. The maximum stress on the bone is at the two ends, so that it is here the bone is expanded with the greatest concentration of trabeculae. The thin, outer shell is the most efficient structure to resist the forces of torque imposed on the bone when this is under twisting and torsional loading, which is exactly what is occuring during flight. See Fig. 6.7. In this situation a thin, hollow cylinder is the most efficient. In consequence of all this, avian bones shatter much more easily during surgery. Except perhaps in very large birds the cortex of avian bones does not form a very sound bed for bone screws. Intramedullary pinning, which in the mammal displaces haemopoetic tissue, in the bird destroys part of the integral strength of the bones.

---

* 'Pseudo monofilament polyamide' (Armour Pharmaceutical Co. Ltd.).

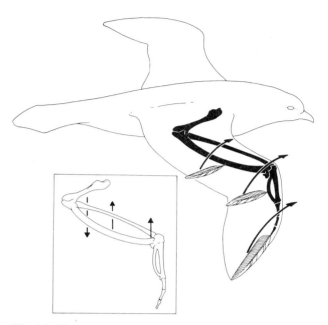

Fig. 6.7. The mechanical forces imposed on the bones of the avian wing during flight. The curved arrows show the torsional stress placed on the bones as the wing descends during flapping flight. The straight arrows illustrate the bending moments applied to the bone at the same time as the torsional stress.

Avian fractures heal in the same manner as those in mammals. This has been demonstrated by Bush, Montali, Novak & James (1976) who showed that fibrous, followed by cartilagenous callus develops from both the peri and endosteal membranes. The rate at which the bone heals is probably a little faster than in mammals. It is most rapid in the smaller birds and one can detect signs of healing on X-ray plates within 8 days. As in mammals, excessive displacement of the fractured ends, movement and infection all retard healing. The so-called very rapid healing of the avian bones reported by a number of workers, may be due to the swift mobilization of fibroblasts and the formation of collagen fibres binding the bones together, rather than complete resolution of the fracture with new bone. Under optimum conditions the gap between the fractured ends is filled with fibrous tissue within 5 days and cancellous bone within 9 days. True boney union takes 22 days and complete remodelling takes 6 weeks.

Apart from the healing of bone, there is little doubt that the maintenance of maximum joint mobility is of far more importance in birds than the attainment of perfect bone alignment. This is not denying that perfectly-aligned bones heal more rapidly.

The pectoral limb

The clavicle

Tiemeier (1941) in a survey of 6212 specimens found 3.41% of wild passeriformes had fractures of the clavicle. These are not often diagnosed by veterinarians and when they are, they are best left alone. It is not practical to splint these bones in any way.

The coracoid

This is a massive bone counteracting the compressive forces of the pectoralis muscle. In a bird of 500 g or more this particular fracture is best dealt with using an intramedullary Steinmann pin. The bone is rather inaccessible, lying deep below the supracoroideus (superficial pectoral) muscle. The muscle needs to be carefully dissected away from the clavicle, the edge of which can be felt subcutaneously at the thoracic inlet (Fig. 6.8). If one half of the fractured coracoid has been displaced inwardly, great care must be taken, in manipulating the bone back into position, because the great vessels from the heart lie just below this region. In small birds the bone will heal by itself and the bird may be able to fly again, but this could take up to one year.

Luxation of the shoulder

The joint is well-supported by muscle and ligament particularly the coraco-humeral ligament. However, the tendon of the supra-coroideus muscle is sometimes stripped from the muscle belly. Rupture of the tendon leads to upward subluxation of the head of the humerus.

The supracoroideus muscle and tendon is best developed in birds with a slow flapping flight, in those which hover and in birds which have a rapid jump take off such as pheasants. In fact, rupture of this tendon has been seen only in pigeons and one crow, both of which have fast-forward flight and in gulls which are mainly gliders.

Surgical approach to the shoulder joint is not difficult. The fibres of the overlying dermatensor muscle are split longitudinally in the

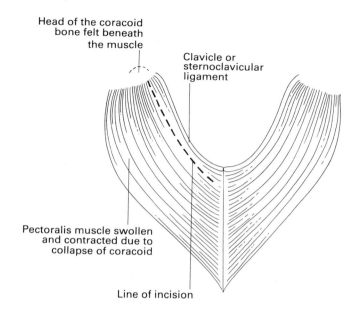

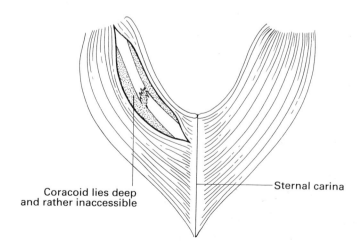

Fig. 6.8. The surgical approach to the coracoid bone.

direction of their fibres and the shoulder joint lies underneath. However, locating and suturing the ruptured tendon back in position is very difficult and an almost impossible task. The retention of complete mobility in the shoulder joint is very important, more so than in any other joint in the wing. All the mechanical forces and differential movements of the wing are concentrated on this joint.

The humerus

The majority of fractures of this bone occur in the middle or at the junction of the middle and lower third of the bone. These are the areas where the bone is least protected by surrounding muscle. In most cases the fractured ends of the bone are well separated and the proximal part is often rotated along its longitudinal axis due to the tension caused by spasm of the contused pectoralis muscle (Fig. 6.9). Although there is an extension of the clavicular air sac into the humerus and damage to this structure can sometimes be seen on X-ray in the region of the pectoralis muscle, it is usually sealed off by blood clot. Emphysema of the tissues is not usually a problem. Since most of the mechanical forces imposed on the wing during flight are transmitted to the humerus it is most important to get accurate alignment and as near perfect resolution of the bone. A slight error in rotational alignment could lead to a change in the angle of attack of the

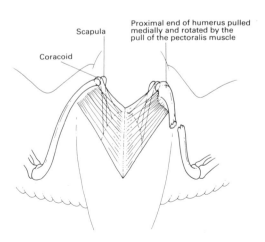

Fig. 6.9. The traction on the proximal end of the fractured humerus by the pectoralis muscle.

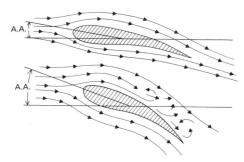

Fig. 6.10. Diagram to illustrate how permanent rotation of the humerus through a badly aligned fracture can affect the angle of attack of the aerofoil section of the wing. The angle of attack (A.A.) affects the airflow across the wing and its lifting qualities.

aerofoil surface and aerodynamic properties of the wing (Fig. 6.10). The bird may well learn to adjust to this situation in time but this only increases its problems of rehabilitation. In spite of all this there are a number of recorded instances in wild birds where the humerus has healed in a grossly distorted position and where the bird has been found flying again. (Olney, 1958/9 ; Tiemeier, 1941).

In a fractured humerus more than 3 days post trauma, and notwithstanding other considerations such as secondary infection, there is always organization in the tissue in response to the trauma. This is more rapid, the smaller the bird. If there is extensive dissection to find and free the bone, there is great risk that the nerves and blood vessels traversing the injured area will be damaged. It is difficult to identify the medullary cavity of a long bone of a small bird in a mass of granulating tissue. If the subject is below 100 grams in weight (cockatiel size) and a captive bird, it may be wiser to leave the fractured wing alone, except to support it with a bandage for 2–3 days (Fig. 6.11). This only needs to be done if the wing is badly dropped and should not be supported for a longer period, which only leads to excessive fibrosis and stiffening of muscles and joints.

On the other hand if the bird is a falcon and is to fly again, some attempt at perfect resolution will have to be made. The avian humerus is well supplied with blood vessels. This has been studied by Jojié & Popovïe (1969) who have shown that there is a separate blood supply to the proximal, middle and distal parts of the humeral shaft. The surgical approach to the bone can be made from either the ventral or dorsal aspect. The latter is probably the easier of the two.

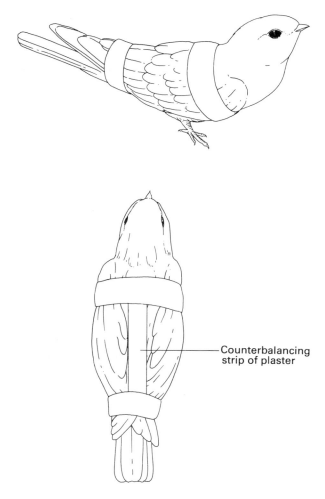

Counterbalancing
strip of plaster

Fig. 6.11. Bandaging the wing of a small bird.

A number of techniques have been devised to repair humeral
fractures.

Intra-medullary pinning

This can be carried out using the standard Steinmann pin and is the
simplest method. In some species such as the goshawk, the humerus is
shaped like an extended 'S' so that it is possible for the ends of the pin

to emerge from the bone away from the shoulder and elbow joints (Fig. 6.12). This is important because any trauma to soft tissues near an avian joint usually leads to excessive fibrosis and reduction in mobility of the joint. Intramedullary pinning also has the disadvantage that it destroys the trabeclar structure of the bone. This will be regenerated when the pin is removed but it does take time. The intramedullary pin does not guard against rotation and, because of the proportionately larger diameter of the avian medullary cavity, a larger and heavier pin has to be used than in a mammal of comparable size. The intramedullary pin does not allow endosteal bone regeneration.

To some extent these disadvantages can be overcome by using one or two smaller diameter pins or Kirschner wire. These may be anchored by a figure-of-eight stainless steel wire through the cortex of the bone above and below the fracture. Place the wire before inserting the pins, after which tighten the wire.

Kirschner splints

This method has been used successfully in large birds by Bush (1981). The pins pass perpendicularly through the skin and cortex of the bone from one side to the other. Four pins are used—two in the proximal half of the bone and two in the distal half. The four pins traversing the bone are then clamped to a rod running parallel to the longitudinal axis of the bone. This is the so called half pin method. If the pins are pushed further through the bone they can be clamped to another pin on the other side of the bone—the full pin technique. The

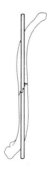

Fig. 6.12. Intramedullary pinning through cortex of curved humerus to avoid the shoulder and elbow joints.

disadvantage of this effective method is weight. The technique is relatively rapid and it does allow endosteal regeneration of the bone.

A modification of this method that is applicable to smaller birds (down to 200 g in size) is to use arthrodesis or Kirschner wires and to anchor these to a piece of plastic (not rubber) tubing filled with methyl methacrylate* based plastic or an epoxy resin glue[†] which then sets and holds the pins firmly. The diameter of the plastic tubing can be adapted to the size of the bird. When the pins need to be removed they are cut through and withdrawn. The advantage of this method is the weight is reduced. Further modification to the technique is to use hypodermic needles placed in predrilled holes and to place the adhesive in the cut off barrel of a 1 ml or 2 ml plastic hypodermic syringe or a trough made from cardboard or an old piece of X-ray film. The pins are held in a mini bone chuck or an instrument maker's chuck. The latter is made of carbon steel and will have to be gas sterilized. when placing the pins in position, the pins farthest apart are first put in position, then joined by the external rod or plastic tube. The bone is aligned and the other pins are placed in position. When using a tube filled with plastic it is sometimes helpful to temporarily anchor the pins to another external pin, parallel to the plastic tube, using wire twisted round the junction. When the whole splint is finished the ends of the pins must be protected, otherwise the bird may be further injured (Fig. 6.13).

Short pin intra medullary devices

The Jonas pin, which is a short pin expanded by a spring when in position, was successfully used by Secord (1958) in repairing fractures on three birds. However, this device is relatively expensive and is unlikely to be readily available in general practice. The author has successfully used short intramedullary pegs made of several materials. These were then held in place by a figure-of-eight stainless wire suture. This method keeps the bone in alignment and helps to put some compression on the fracture site to aid healing (Fig. 6.14). The materials used for the intramedullary pegs have ranged from short lengths of a Steinmann pin, cut-off and smoothed 18 to 4 gauge hypodermic needles, carbon fibre rods and polypropamide rods. The

---

* 'Technovit 6091' (Kulzer & Co. GmbH.).
[†] 'Araldyte' (Ciba Geigy).

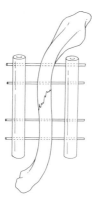

Fig. 6.13. Method of internal splinting a fractured bone using the Kirschner type splint made from Kirschner wire and the barrels of 1 ml hypodermic plastic syringes filled with glue. Leave enough space to enable the pins to be cut when the splint is removed.

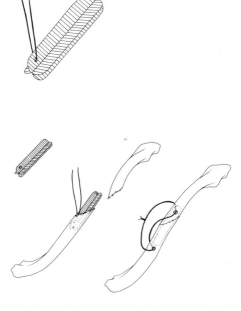

Fig. 6.14. The method of using a peg made of crucate section plastic and a figure-of-eight wire suture to reduce a fractured humerus.

latter were obtained by using the plunger stem of a plastic hypodermic syringe. The stem is cut to approximate size and then cut down and filed to shape during the operation using a sterile file. The material snaps if too long a length is used, but only a short peg is needed to hold the bone in alignment. If the fracture is more than a few days old the medullary cavity will have to be reamed out of new endosteal bone. The peg is pushed into the longer fragment first and then reversed into the shorter piece of the bone. The reversal is accomplished by pulling on a piece of suture material threaded through a hole drilled at the end of the peg. Holes for the tension band sutures are then drilled with a fine drill bit or a straight triangular needle. This can be held in a mini bone chuck or an instrument maker's chuck and rotated between the fingers. One hole may go through the intramedullary peg but the other hole must be beyond the end of the peg, otherwise the bone cannot be pulled together. Too much tension must not be put on the wire suture, the fragments must be carefully brought together to avoid splitting (Fig. 6.13). When passing the wire suture through the drill holes it is sometimes useful to use a hypodermic needle as a wire guide.

The method can be tedious but it does allow some endosteal bone formation as the peg has a cruciate cross section. It is also light in weight and the polypropamide is well-tolerated.

Unfortunaely many humeral fractures are compound and grossly contaminated. Osteomyelitis does not affect birds systemically so much as mammals but it prevents healing. Bacteriological culture for antibiotic sensitivity should always be carried out. A variety of organisms have been isolated but coliform organisms are common.

The whole area should be cleaned and debrided. If the bone is discoloured and necrotic it is best removed, even if this means a reduction in the length of the bone. Provided not more than 25% of the length of the bone is lost some birds will learn to adapt and may even fly again, (Olney, 1958/9); (Scott, 1968).

After operating on the humerus the wing is best strapped in the folded position to the body for 2–3 days (Fig. 6.15). This short period of bandaging should not be extended because the circulation is restricted. Low oxygen tension in traumatized tissue probably predisposes the tissue to excessive fibrosis. A suitable perch should be provided to stop the primary feathers trailing on the floor.

Atrophy of muscle through disuse can be rapid in birds. The white muscle fibres (the glycogen users) as distinct from the red muscle

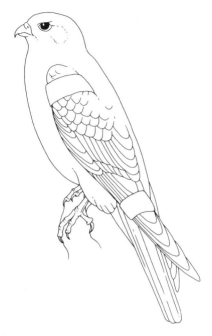

Fig. 6.15. Bandaging the wing of a large bird.

fibres (the fat users) are more susceptible to atrophy when subject to disuse (George & Berger, 1978). There is always a mixture of the two types of fibres in the pectoralis muscle of all birds but the proportion varies with the species. Birds that have a rapid jump take off, such as pheasants, have a higher proportion of white fibres so the chances of disuse atrophy in the pectoralis of these species is higher.

Luxation of the elbow joint

This is not uncommon and can be an intractable. The joint is covered by a weak joint capsule—common to humerus, radius and ulna. There is little surrounding muscle to give protection. Any attempt to stabilize the joint with wire sutures is quite likely to end in fibrosis and even eventual ankylosis. A hinged splint is required in order that the bones are kept in place while the joint can continue to function. Rodger (J.L. 1981; personal communication) used this method successfully on a buzzard. A strip of aluminium padded 'finger' splint bent over the olecranon and sutured in position, using holes drilled through the aluminium, may work. The sutures pass through the skin, anterior and posterior to the ulna and between the shafts of the secondary feathers. When attempting to relocate the displaced bones, the covert feathers should be plucked and the whole are wetted so that the anatomy of the parts can be seen.

Fractures of the radius and ulna

In about 50% of cases either the radius or the ulna is fractured, but not both. When only one bone is fractured it is wiser to leave the fractured bone alone. The normal one will help to splint it. Even if there is not perfect alignment of the healed fractured bone this does not matter, the bird will manage quite adequately and fly again. Strapping of the wing for 2–3 days only is required (see earlier note on pages 149 and 154). If both radius and ulna are fractured some method of splinting will be required.

External splinting

This is more applicable to the smaller birds where the bones may not be thick enough to support some method of internal fixation. One type of external splint is to suture a piece of lightweight plastic material such as a length of 'Hexcelite'* or 'Vetcast casting tape'† padded with polyurethane foam over the fracture site. The sutures pass through the mesh of the splinting material through the skin and between the shafts of the secondary feathers (Fig. 6.16). It is best to remove most of the covert feathers and to wet the area so that the anatomy of the parts can be distinguished through the semi-transparent skin. The sutures should be placed well behind the ulna so that the main blood vessels are avoided. However, if possible, the posterior sutures should be placed in front of the interremigial ligament. All the sutures should be preplaced before being tied so that they can be accurately positioned (Fig. 6.16). This splint is light in weight, is comfortable, and, providing it is properly positioned, does allow some movement of the joints during healing. A similar type but simpler splint, using X-ray film, is applicable to birds the size of a canary (20 g) and is described under fractures of the carpus.

* (Hexcel Medical Products).
† (Animal Care Products).

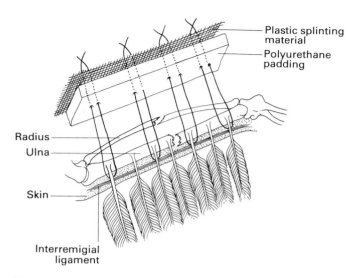

Plastic splinting
material

Polyurethane
padding

Radius

Ulna

Skin

Interremigial
ligament

Fig. 6.16. Method of external splinting of the fractured ulna using a mesh of plastic splinting material.

Internal splinting

The Kirschner splint as described for use in fractures of the humerus is quite applicable to fractures of radius and ulna.

The author also once used the barrel of a 1 ml plastic tuberculin syringe cut to size and smoothed off at the ends. This was used as a sleeve to push over the outside of the fractured ulna of a barn owl. A cut was made along the posterior side of this cylinder so that it would slide past the shafts of the adjacent secondary feathers, which are directly attached to the bone. This prosthetic sleeve was sufficiently firm when in position so that no further anchorage was necessary. This provided excellent alignment and the bird was able to fly perfectly with the sleeve permanently in position.

Fractures of the carpus, metacarpus and digits

In very large birds it is possible to use a Kirschner Emmer splint, but in birds below 2 kg in weight the metacarpal bone is so thin the method is not practical. A method of external splinting that the author has found to work quite well is to use a piece of disused X-ray film or clear acetate sheet. This is bent over the leading edge of the wing and held in position by sutures. The sutures pass through the skin covering the primary feathers. Just posterior to the carpus and metacarpus is the ulnocarporemigial aponeurosis (King & McLelland, 1984a). This triangular aponeurotic sheet gives very good anchorage for the sutures (Fig. 6.17). This splint is light in weight and allows some movement of the carpal joint. Many medium sized birds (200 g – 1 kg) on which this splint has been used have been able to fly again.

In very small birds suturing the shafts of the adjacent primary feathers together on each side of the fracture may work—as the shafts are directly attached to the bone.

Pinioning and wing feather cutting

The practitioner is sometimes asked to carry out these procedures on free ranging birds to stop them flying. Amputation of the tip of the wing may be required in those birds that sometimes suffer from a so-called 'slipped wing' (see Chapter 1, p. 16). Simple cutting short of the primary and possibly some of the secondary feathers will also prevent flight. A sharp pair of strong scissors is sufficient for the operation, and providing the shaft is cut whilst the feather is not growing (i.e. not in their 'pins'), it does not bleed. It is best to leave the outer one or two primaries which will cover the defect in the wing when it is folded and lead to a better cosmetic appearance. Only one wing is treated since the principle is to unbalance the bird's flight. If both wings are operated on, many birds are able to achieve short distance flight, certainly over an enclosure fence.

Amputation of the wing tip for pinioning is carried out through the 3rd and 6th metacarpal bones, just distal to the carpus. The blood

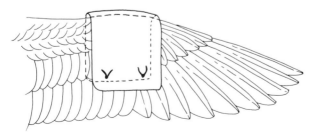

Fig. 6.17. Method of external splinting of the carpus and metacarpus using acetate film.

supply to this area, particularly when the feathers are growing, can be well developed. It is therefore wise to place a tourniquet around the carpal area just proximal to the attachment of the 2nd metacarpal or alula digit (attachment of bastard wing) before making any incision. If the covert feathers are well-plucked from the area and the operation site is wet, the underlying structures can more easily be seen. An encircling incision is made through the skin at least half way along the length of the 3rd and 4th metacarpal bones, so that there is plenty of skin left to cover the ends of the bone. The skin, tendons and any muscle is then dissected back to the proximal end of the 3rd and 4th metacarpal bones. These are cut at this level with bone forceps or strong scissors (Fig. 6.18). If the temporary ligature is effective, bleeding is minimal, otherwise there can be a lot of haemorrhage which is difficult to control. The skin and other soft tissue is then sutured so that the remaining muscle will cover the ends of the bone.

Patagiectomy

This operation, devised by Mangili (1971) and later used by Robinson (1975) is to render large birds flightless. It can also be used in some cases where a wing is so badly injured that amputation is considered necessary. The end result is not only cosmetically more acceptable than amputation but may well enable the bird to maintain better balance. The technique is illustrated in Fig. 6.19.

Tenotomy of the extensor tendons on the cranial edge of the metacarpal bone has been used to deflight birds as well as wiring the carpal bones together.

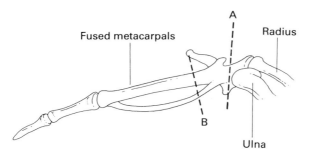

Fig. 6.18. Pinioning of the wing. A, Position of the tourniquet; B, Position of amputation.

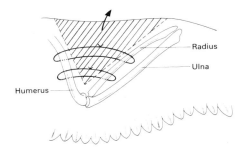

Fig. 6.19. Patagiectomy. The shaded area of the prepatagium is removed after each side is clamped with artery forceps and the area is closed by sutures placed around the humerus and radius. The edges of the skin on the dorsal and ventral surfaces are sutured.

The pelvic limb

Fractures of the femur and the tibio tarsal bone

These can all be dealt with by one of the methods described for internal fixation of the fractured humerus. The surgical approach to both these bones is from the lateral aspect and is not difficult so long as the muscles are carefully dissected apart and split in the direction of their muscle fibres.

In the case of the tibio tarsal bone with a transverse midshaft fracture there is a definite tendency for the distal end of the bone to rotate outwardly. Whilst this is often not a problem to the bird, which often manages quite well, it is usually not acceptable to the owner. The rotation is probably caused by the tension of the digital flexor muscles involved in the perching mechanism. This is one reason why intramedullary pinning of the tibio tarsal bone is often not entirely satisfactory.

Because of the conical shape of the muscles surrounding the tibio tarsal bone, external splinting is not well adapted to this area.

Fractures of the bones below the hock joint

Except in the case of the larger birds, where Kirschner Emmer-splinting is very suitable to fractures of these bones, external splinting often produces good results. In birds over 100 g (cockatiel) in weight a plastic splinting material such as 'Hexcelite'* or 'Vetcast tape'[†], padded with a 5–6 mm thick piece of expanded polyurethane, works very well. The polyurethane pad is cut generously so that it overlaps the area to be splinted. When the softened Hexcelite is placed in position it is moulded to the part by binding snugly with an elastic bandage such as 'Vetrap'[†]. The excess polyurethane padding and any sharp projections of Hexcelite can be trimmed with scissors.

In small birds like budgerigars and canaries—up to cockatiel size, the use of a splint made of a strip of sticking plaster has been described by a number of authors and is very effective. Any tape material that sticks to itself is effective, but zinc oxide plaster is probably the best. The application of the splint is illustrated in Fig. 6.20 and it can be reinforced by incorporating match sticks, cocktail sticks, nylon catheter tubing, etc., within the layers of the splint. When applying these external splints, they can always be placed much more effectively if the bird is under light anaesthesia. This allows muscle relaxation and better alignment. Trying to fit a splint on a struggling, conscious bird may result in further trauma.

A few birds will not tolerate the splint and remove it in a few days. Even if the splint is only in place for about 4 days it has often been found to be sufficient time in these very small birds.

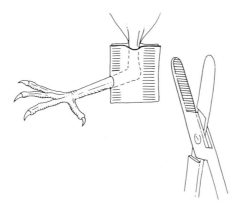

Fig. 6.20. Splint for small birds using adhesive tape crimped together with artery forceps.

* (Hexcel Medical Products).
[†] (Animal Care Products).

When the time comes for removal of the splint, soaking the zinc oxide splint in ether or other solvent* will dissolve the adhesive. Again it is safer to carry this out if the bird is under light anaesthesia.

The removal of rings around the tarso metatarsal bone

In budgerigars, particularly, but also in other birds it is often necessary to remove a metal identification ring. The ring may have excoriated the underlying scales, or worse, the underlying tissue may have begun to swell, so that the ring acts as a ligature causing swelling of the whole foot. If this is not promptly relieved the blood supply can be cut off and the foot becomes gangrenous. Very often the ring has become buried in the inflamed and swollen tissues by the time veterinary advice is sought. It is most important to have the bird held firmly on a table by another person. General anaesthesia may be necessary. The surgeon can then hold the ring firmly with artery forceps whilst the ring is cut with the points of a pair of nail clippers. There is a risk that the ring will slip out of the grip of the artery forceps and rotate whilst being cut. Great care must be taken to avoid this otherwise the tibio tarsus may be fractured. Specially designed cutters are available for this purpose.

Bumblefoot

This is a septic condition of the foot leading to abscessation. It has been recognized in poultry for years and is not uncommon amongst falconers' birds. It is also seen in water birds and occasionally even in budgerigars. It is a serious condition and can ruin a bird for falconry. It is rarely, if ever, seen in wild birds. The infection penetrates the foot from the plantar surface because the integrity of the integument has been impaired. This can take place in water birds if the feet become excessively dry or the skin is abraded. Falcons and heavy, inactive birds, constantly standing on the same diameter perches so that their feet get little exercise are predisposed to bumblefoot. Cooper (1978) discusses the subject thoroughly in his book and points out that puncture of the metatarsal pad or sole by an overgrown claw of the first or hind digit may cause this condition in some falcons.

* Available from pharmacists.

The feet of birds are covered with scales which are modified areas of the epidermis. The scales are formed by areas of hyperkeratinazation. Between them are sulci or clefts. Some areas of the feet are raised in papillae which increases the grip of the foot. There is constant growth and shedding of the skin surface through normal wear. Sometimes the scales are shed during the moult of the feathers. Anything that interferes with this normal pattern of skin change, such as excessive abrasion, will allow micro-organisms to reach the subdermal tissues. Any bird kept in dirty, unhygienic conditions is subject to bumblefoot. The skin is tight and in places adherent to the underlying bone. Any swelling in this region due to an inflammatory response is restricted and tends to tract along tendon sheaths and other planes of least resistance. Within a few days of the initial infection, fibroplasia sets in—possibly exacerbated by a low oxygen tension through swelling of the tissues and inactivity of the sessile, tethered falcon. The increased fibrous tissue retards any penetration of antibodies to the focus of infection. The whole process is a vicious circle. The abscess may be filled with caseous or sero sanguinous pus and may contain a variety of micro-organisms. These commonly include staphlococcus aureus, *Escherichia coli* and proteus species. The infection may track as far as the intertarsal or hock joint. when first presented for veterinary examination the lesion may be 3–4 months old or even longer. The obvious swelling is usually covered by a scab caused by hyperkeratinization. The foot should be X-rayed in the lateral and dorsal ventral positions because osteoarthritis is a common sequel to a long standing infection. The scab should be removed and a bacteriological culture taken for antibiotic sensitivity. Swelling of the tendon sheaths and teno sinovitis can sometimes be detected because when the digits are moved under general anaesthesia small ratchet-like projections on the inside of the tendon sheaths catch with those on the tendons, making the movement feel jerky. This ratchet mechanism is normally brought into play when the bird is perching and there is tension on the flexor tendons. In the relaxed anaesthetised bird there should be no tension on these tendons.

If the swelling on the foot is very small and there is no sign of the infection tracking, it may be treated with the appropriate systemic and local antibiotics. The local antibiotics may be mixed with dimethyl sulphoxide* to help penetration of the drugs. Vitamin A

---

* 'Demavet' (E.R. Squibb & Sons Ltd.).

given systemically may help improve the health of the integument.

In the vast majority of cases surgery will be necessary. This consists of opening the abscess and carefully removing all caseous and necrotic material, taking care to avoid nerves, tendons and blood vessels. All sinuses should be investigated with a blunt probe and the whole area should be vigorously irrigated, preferably with trypsin solution. Before starting it is a wise precaution to place a tourniquet around the lower part of the tibio tarsal bone because the granulating tissue within the swelling can bleed profusely. The tourniquet should be released periodically. After thorough curettage the skin is sutured with mattress sutures using non-absorbable suture material, preferably placed across the line of flexion of the skin. The foot is bandaged and the bandage may be left in place 2–3 weeks until healing is completed. A non-adhesive dressing such as fucidin intertulle should be placed under the bandage. The bird should be allowed onto a perch padded with foam rubber or plastic foam. The patient should be encouraged to use a variety of different sized and shaped perches so that the foot is not constantly held in the same position. The perches may need to be permanently padded and very strict attention to hygiene must be the rule. The owner should be constantly aware of the problem and routinely examine the feet for the early signs of trouble.

7 / Nursing and After-Care

This chapter is based on a paper by the author published in the *Journal of Small Animal Practice* (1984) **25**, 275–288. Sections of it are reprinted here by permission of the editor and publishers.

Many practices have an appreciable small animal clientele and are already well-equipped with trained nursing staff and facilities for hospitalizing cats and dogs and also increasingly for the smaller, children's pets. However, few practices routinely hospitalize birds. This is regrettable because, apart from wild bird casualties for which the public expects immediate expert veterinary attention, diagnosis in individually owned birds is difficult. A practice routine for hospitalizing more avian patients will give the veterinarian time to observe and evaluate the bird, leading to a more accurate diagnosis and a higher standard of treatment.

Hospitalizing birds is also advantageous to nursing staff. The clinical state of avian patients can change hourly, often with little obvious signs. Nurses, developing their ability to recognize these slight changes, enhance their powers of observation of all patients, and because of the delicate nature of many sick birds, proficiency acquired in nursing these creatures leads to a general upgrading of all nursing skills.

The essential attributes that are common in all branches of nursing are (a) a diligent attention to hygiene, (b) a genuine concern for the well-being of the patient, (c) accurate recording of the clinical progress, and (d) a methodical approach to the task in hand.

Many of the techniques and skills used by the veterinary clinician and the animal nurse have been developed and adapted from those used in human nursing. However, there are dangers in the extrapolation of knowledge from one branch of science to another.

Successful avian nursing depends on the realization that there are fundamental differences in the biology of birds and mammals.

Aspects of bird behaviour influencing avian nursing

Reduction of stress

When hospitalized, birds are generally more liable to psychological stress than mammals. Bird behaviour is largely instinctive. A routine behavioural response is triggered by a specific stimulus or releaser present in the environment. If there are none of the normal releasers in the bird's hospital environment the creature becomes stressed. Similarly, a bird will make certain ritualistic movements that act as greetings, threats, etc. to a member of its own species. If the bird makes these to its human handler and there is no response it becomes stressed. Stress is also related to birds' high metabolic rates and to the fact that most birds are creatures of the air and less used to confined surroundings. Stress, caused by fright or frustration of confinement, will vary among species and be influenced by their degree of habituation to man. Even within species there is considerable variation. Some wild barn owls (*Tyto alba*), for example, willingly eat dead hatchery chicks whilst others have to be persuaded to do so—this being quite unrelated to the severity of their injuries. Most hospitalized parrots will feed readily, but occasionally one will sulk and feed only on one part of its normal diet (e.g. hemp) for which it has a particular liking.

Aviculturalists recognize that some birds will feed out of, for example, a red dish which they are used to, but will not touch a blue dish of exactly the same type. Some kestrels (*Falco tinnunculus*) are more agressive than others. Apart from individual differences within a species, some types of bird are more easily handled than others. Amongst raptors, buzzards (*Buteo buteo*) are generally much less agressive than goshawks (*Accipiter gentilis*) or sparrow hawks (*Accipiter nisus*).

However, there are some aspects of avian behaviour that are common to all birds with relatively few exceptions. With the exclusion of the ground-living species such as fowls (Galliformes) and waterfowl (Anseriformes), most birds spend a great deal of their time above human eye-level—either in flight or perching. Consequently, when hospitalized, birds are less stressed if they are kept at as high a level as is practical in a room. Their cages, if portable, can be kept on a high shelf. In contrast to this, if one is feeding altricial nestlings, these creatures inherently expect a parent bird bringing food to approach from above. If the nurse is to simulate this pattern of behaviour the chick must be approached from above not from a horizontal direction.

Although all birds have good hearing, abnormal sounds, such as a nearby human voice or barking of a hospitalized dog, seem to disturb them much less than the sight of, or quick movement of, other creatures. This is particularly so with wild birds which are not accustomed to human contact. The nurse must learn to move slowly and deliberately when in the bird's vicinity. Ideally, hospitalized birds are less stressed if kept in a separate room out of sight and sound of creatures other than birds, where the light intensity can be suitably reduced and where higher ambient temperatures can be maintained. However, in most veterinary hospitals this is not practical because of the other patients and a compromise has to be reached. A reduced light level is most easily achieved by putting a blanket or dark cloth over the cage and in some cases providing the bird with a box or nest compartment in which to hide. A blanket across the front of the cage will sometimes stop a bird continually bouncing the bars of its cage and so causing self-inflicted injury. Nevertheless, care must be taken not to restrict the ventilation or indeed, to restrict the nurse's constant vigilance of the patient. If birds are frequently hospitalized, a thin board, covered in easily cleaned plastic laminte, can be made to hang across the front of the cage. This board can also be used when cleaning out the cage so as to confine the bird to one corner without actually handling it. There is less disturbance to the bird if the cage has a removable tray, similar to those provided in the common type of budgerigar or parrot cage.

When hospitalizing dogs, or dogs and cats in a mixed animal hospital ward, it is usual not to have the cages facing each other. This reduces barking and the stress of animal patients and nursing staff. With birds it is often better to let the birds see each other, particularly in the case of social species. Birds often live in flocks of the same or allied species. Some birds, such as hospitalized psittacines, may have led a long, solitary caged existence and sometimes seem to derive benefit from seeing or being near another similar bird. In the budgerigar this is particularly noticeable. A bird that was relatively inactive will suddenly become more alert and interested in its environment. Some parrots will sometimes reduce or cease self-plucking of their feathers.

The one type of bird that all species instinctively recognize is the predator. If hospitalized, this type of bird must be kept out of sight of other birds. Even parrots will recognize and fluff up their plumage if they see a peregrine falcon which does not occur in their country of origin. Hospitalized raptors are usually silent so that other birds do not know they are in the same room unless they see them.

Perches

Many of the birds that veterinarians treat use perches. There is little doubt this type of bird, confined to a cage, is much happier and less stressed if it has somewhere to perch. This instinct in some birds is so strong that even those born with feet so deformed that they are unable to grip will still attempt to perch using the sides of their feet. Ideally there should be more than one perch and these should be of varying size and surface texture so that the muscles of the feet are constantly exercised and do not become cramped. The standard perch used by aviculturalists is made of a round wooden dowel and, although easy to keep clean, it is not really ideal because of its uniform diameter and smooth surface. Natural twigs or branches are better and can be replaced when dirty and worn. Branches from most deciduous trees (except oak) can be used, but those from rhododendron and yew are best avoided when used for psittaccines—which like to gnaw. For medium to large birds weighing 200 g to 1500 g, a robust, temporary block perch can be utilized from a brick or an earthenware flowerpot turned upside down. This can be covered with a piece of cloth. A block of wood covered with soft leather makes an even better perch. These coverings need replacement or cleaning when dirty but they provide a good grip and protection from abrasion which predisposes to infection of the feet, and to which birds are prone. All perches should be high enough to prevent the plumage of the birds trailing on the floor—where it is liable to become frayed and soiled. In hospitalized birds, tail feathers can be protected from fraying and damage if bound with a water-soluble, gummed paper tape. Wooden perches can be replaced across the corner of the cages since some birds, such as owls, like to lean against the side of the cage when roosting. Perches should be placed so that when the bird defecates the droppings do not contaminate the food or water containers, or fall on another bird beneath it. The faeces of some falcons are ejected horizontally instead of dropping vertically.

Bathing

Most birds bathe more frequently than most mammals, and many raptors, including owls, will bathe if given the opportunity. Aviculturalists recognize this, and many of them regularly spray their show birds with a fine mist of water from a spray. Aviary birds can be sprayed with a fine jet from a garden hose. When this is done, birds will purposefully fly into the spray, just as aviary birds will deliberately go out into rain. Falconers put their birds out, tethered to a perch, to weather and offer them regular baths. Consequently, whenever it is practical and when not inconsistent with other veterinary treatment, hospitalized birds will benefit if given a bath or sprayed with a fine mist from a household spray. The depth of water in a bird bath should not be more than half an inch for small birds and not more than one inch for a bird the size of a tawny owl (*Strix aluco*), otherwise there is a risk of drowning. Chicks should not be bathed, since in many species the down does not give them sufficient protection.

Because of the desire of most birds to bathe, their drinking water containers should not be too large and should generally be kept above ground level. The temperature of the water used for bathing should be about 104°F (40°C). Bathing keeps the plumage clean and also encourages active preening. This is a normal activity of the healthy bird, since the maintenance of the plumage is not only essential for flight but also for the conservation of body temperature. In waterfowl (Anseriformes) and in gulls and waders (Charadriiformes) the skin of the feet needs constant contact with water to remain healthy, otherwise ulceration and infection may develop. In the Anseriformes, putting the bird into the water of a bath may also act as the releaser to start it preening.

The advantages and disadvantages of constant handling

Tender loving care by the nurse is of particular benefit to nestlings before their eyes open and will also benefit all ages of birds used to human contact. McKeever (1979) suggests that with baby owls, a piece of dark cloth hung over the top of their box, or a soft toy to nestle up to will be beneficial and simulate physical contact with the adult bird or with the young birds' siblings.

Too much handling and attention can be disadvantageous to an adult wild bird because the creature becomes tame and this may be a danger if release is intended. However, if the bird is to be regularly handled for medical treatment then the sooner it gets conditioned to human contact the better.

Physiological considerations when nursing birds

The implications of a high metabolic rate

Energy requirements

The animal nurse regularly nursing dogs and cats must be aware that birds have a higher basal metabolic rate. This is directly related to the fact that the body surface area to body volume ratio increases with decreasing body weight. All birds tend to look larger than they really are because the depth of plumage, holding insulating static air in contact with the skin, is thicker than the corresponding layer of hair covering most mammals of comparable size. However, Kendeigh (1970) has indicated that there are other factors, such as the weight of feathers per unit of surface area and the microscopic anatomy and physiology of body organs, which influence the rate of metabolism. Also basal metabolic rate is higher in passerines compared with nonpasserines (Lasiewski & Dawson, 1967). High rates of metabolism mean rapid heat loss and rapid utilization of the body's energy reserves of glycogen and fat. This is so marked that birds will regularly and normally lose weight overnight whilst they are not feeding (Perrins, 1979). This is particularly marked if the ambient temperature is low e.g. 30°F (-1°C). Consequently, healthy birds of the order of 10 g bodyweight e.g. blue tits (*Parus caeruleus*), kept under optimum conditions of minimal stress, minimal activity and an ambient temperature of 60°F (15.5°C) probably cannot survive more than 48 to 72 hours without food. As size increases, survival from inanition will be longer. Food intake in hospitalized small birds needs to be frequent. If the bird is not feeding itself, nourishment needs to be given at least every hour. Feeding two or three times daily as for small hospitalized mammals is just not sufficient. Small healthy birds need of the order of 1 k cal of energy per gram of bodyweight (Perrins, 1979). One gram of fat yields about 9 kg calories and 1 kg of carbohydrate yields about 4 kg calories. A 20 g canary therefore needs to take in about 5 g of utilizable carbohydrate a day or approximately half this quantity of lipids. Perrins (1979) pointed out that great tits (*Parus major*) feed nestlings between 58 and 78 times daily. Very small birds of 20 g and below this weight which have lost condition through illness, need the maximum number of daylight hours in which to feed. It is a wise precaution with these small birds to leave the animal room lights on throughout the night, particularly during the winter months. In larger birds, particularly raptors, the feeding requirements are not quite so stringent. It is reasonable to feed these birds once or twice daily and, provided the food intake is regular, they can with advantage go without food one day a week. The work of Kirkwood (1981) has done much to clarify the rate at which weight is lost in raptors during starvation.

Effect of the inflammatory response

The basal metabolic rate of all homoiotherms increases as part of the body's inflammatory response to disease. This leads to even greater energy demands and a more rapid loss of weight mediated by a complex neuron-endocrine response (Richards, 1980). The nurse should be constantly monitoring the condition of a sick bird by palpation of its pectoral muscles and, where practical, by weighing the bird daily using the methods described on p. 59. Variation in weight is one of the most reliable and easily measurable parameters in a bird's daily progress. The nurse will need to use discretion regarding how much stress is caused to the individual bird by weighing and should not carry this out if the bird gets too excited. As a consequence of an increased metabolic rate, tissues probably heal more quickly. Also irreversible pathological changes, such as fibrosis and the formation of scar tissue in traumatized muscle, takes place more rapidly in small birds than in mammals.

Ambient temperature

To maintain a high rate of metabolism, the normal body temperature of all birds is about 105°F (40°C) and in very small birds, particularly passerines it may reach 107°F (41°C). There may be a diurnal variation of 4–5°F (2–3°C). All sick and severely injured birds, which are rapidly depleting their limited energy reserves, will be less stressed if their environmental temperature is raised to at least 80°F (26°C). Sometimes this can, with benefit, be increased to 100°F (37.7°C) for a period of 24 to 48 hours, after which it is gradually reduced. In many veterinary practices warmth will be administered using an infrared lamp. It will be better if this is controlled by an ordinary household dimmer switch; alternatively, the lamp can be gradually moved further away. As with animals, it is essential that the lamp is not too close and that the bird is able to get away from the direct beam. A hot water bottle wrapped in newspaper and placed together with the patient in a cardboard box with ventilation holes in the top of the box will provide warmth in an emergency situation.

It should be remembered that oiled birds have lost their normal insulation and need emergency protection from heat loss.

Special bird hospital cages are available commercially in which the temperature of the cage can be controlled thermostatically. However, the thermostats in these cages may not be very sensitive. Also, these cages often do not have any means of controlling humidity and, because the volume of the cage is relatively small, they need to be well ventilated without actually creating a draught. Probably the best means to achieve a high degree of control over temperature and humidity is the use of a premature baby incubator. These have a facility for enriching the air supply with oxygen and controlling humidity. Incubators need to be adequately ventilated to reduce the risk of infective organisms from dried faecal matter and other body excreta being inhaled by the bird. Incubators are a potent source of infection and need to be kept scrupulously clean.

The physiological consequences of the avian air sac system

As mentioned on p. 68 the air sacs are prone to infection. This is exacerbated in the resting bird because flying activity and, in particular, the action of the main flight muscles alternatively contracting and relaxing, helps to pump air through the air sacs and at the same time cooling the hard working muscle. The continual forceful flushing of air through the air sac system reduces the chances of pathogenic organisms contained in this warm, moist, internal atmosphere of establishing themselves on the surface of the air sac.

Because of the large internal surface area of the air sacs and high body temperature, small birds have an inherently high water loss from the pulmonary system. Many small birds obtain a lot of their water requirements from metabolized food and body fat stores. Therefore all sick or injured birds that have not been feeding can be assumed to be dehydrated.

Dehydration in birds

Dehydrated birds should be given fluid either by mouth or by subcutaneous injection. The injection of fluid can be made over the pectoral muscles, in the propatagial skin fold of the wing, inside the thigh, or at the base of the neck. Redig (1979) recommends using a 5% glucose saline solution; this given at the rate of 4% of the body weight divided into two or three doses daily. This volume needs to be halved for small birds, and Steiner & Davis (1981) recommend using 0.1$^{\#}$ml of Hartmann's solution every 10–15 minutes in the budgerigar, using alternate sides of the body. The rate of absorption is increased if hyaluronidase is added to the fluid.

Extreme care must be taken in giving subcutaneous injections in birds since avian skin in not as elastic as mammalian skin and aqueous injections tend to ooze out through the needle puncture if too much is given at one site.

As a consequence of the usual dehydration in sick and injured birds, constipation easily occurs. Johnson (1979) states that the rectum and coprodaeum are areas of active water absorption, and reflux passage of fluid contents (urine and faeces) occurs from these areas as far as, and into the caeca. Other considerations apart, dehydration will lead to the cessation of these physiological activities and devitalization of the associated tissues, resulting in constipation. McKeever (1979) suggests relieving this condition by manual evacuation; the use of a warm saline enema is sometime useful.

Feeding hospitalized birds

There is little problem with birds that are eating. The owner of an exotic cage or aviary bird or the owner of a falcon will be pleased to advise on what to feed, and will often supply suitable food. However, if a falconer's sick bird is received into the hospital, the nurse should be made aware that these birds are sometimes kept short of food by their owners to make them keen hunters, and sick or injured raptors under stress may be near starvation. Wild birds may not have been feeding for sometime before being found. The main problems for the nurse arise with the nutrition of the emergency case which cannot, or will not feed readily, or in the case of the wild bird, for which there is none of the normal diet readily to hand. As a rule, a 10% solution of glucose or glucose saline given by mouth at the rate of 10 ml/kg body weight will help. However, it needs to be given at least once every half hour, but even then it will not meet the daily maintenance requirements of metabolizable energy. If this is supplemented, at the same rate, with a protein hydrolysate preparation (e.g. Ovigest* or Lamb Tonic[†]) the bird may be kept alive for a little longer. Preparations containing amino-acids and essential vitamins are better (e.g. Duphalyte[‡]) since they provide a more comprehensive range of nutrients. These can be given subcutaneously in quantities similar to those given for fluid therapy.

Other artifical feeds made for human invalids and infants (e.g. Complan,[§] Build-up,[¶] Vita food,[**] and Farlene[§]) are useful. They contain fairly high levels of energy-yielding constituents, mainly in the form of carbohydrates with some vegetable fats. All these artificial foods contain about 4 g calories per gram of food. A small bird weighing 20 g requires at least 5 g per day of these foods to maintain its requirements. Their digestibility is improved if the contents of a Pancrex V[††] capsule is mixed with the food prior to administration.

All these invalid and infant foods can be given in a liquid form with the aid of a stomach tube—an easy task, because of the large diameter of the avian oropharynx and oesophagus. The stomach tube must be placed well down into the oesophagus or crop of the bird. Stomach tubes can be devised from suitable diameter pieces of rubber or plastic tubing fitted to the nozzle of a plastic syringe. One can also use a rigid metal stomach catheter if this is well-lubricated and allowed to slip into the oesophagus under its own weight. When the bird's head and neck are extended in a vertical direction, there is little danger of tramua. However, one must be careful not to force the tube down the oesophagus. When passing a stomach tube the progress of this tube can often be seen particularly in a long necked bird like a swan, as it passes down the dorsal aspect of the neck. It passes under the trachea just before the thoracic inlet.

Another type of preparation that can be used for the general feeding

* Ovigest; (Welcome).
[†] Lamb Tonic; (Crown Chemical Co. Ltd).
[‡] Duphalyte; (Duphar Veterinary Ltd).
[§] Complan and Farlene; (Farley Health Foods Ltd).
[¶] Build-up; (Carnation Foods Ltd).
** Vita food; (Boots PLC).
[††] Pancrex V; (Paines & Byrne Ltd).

of sick birds is Convalescent Diet* which is specially formulated for invalid dogs and cats. These foods are of animal origin and are designed for carnivores. Except for some very specialized feeders,—frugivorous species for example, humming birds and sunbirds, all species of birds are probably capable of digesting this type of food. These foods are soft and can be forced into the barrel of a 2 ml plastic syringe so that when the plunger is depressed the food is extruded from the nozzle as a small worm-like thread which some birds will readily pick at. Another method of administering semi-solid foods is to cut off the nozzle of the 2 ml syringe to enlarge the orifice and then place a plug of the food into the bird's oropharynx. Care must be taken to place the food well beyond the glottis, which in most birds is on the floor of the mouth just behind the root of the tongue. In some birds such as the heron (*Ardea cinerea*) it may be farther back.

A food that is suitable for most species of orphan birds, as well as invalid birds, is mashed, hard boiled, or scrambled eggs mixed with an equal quantity of sweet biscuit meal, or bread crumbs, with a little glucose powder added. This mixture should be slightly moistened and can be given by one of the above methods. If given too dry, the food is not easily swallowed. This mixture can also be offered to small nestlings on the tip of an artist's brush. Some aviculturalists feeding parrot nestlings use a small spoon bent up at the tip to form a sort of scoop shaped like the mandible of a parent bird.

All these foods require less mechanical work by the bird's alimentary canal and so a more rapid and economical utilization takes place.

Once the initial emergency period of convalescence has passed, the nurse should consider providing food for the patient which is as near to its normal diet as possible. Start by adding 5% glucose to the bird's normal diet and liquidizing this in a food blender—this aids digestion. Birds are very specialized feeders with varied adaptations of their anatomy for this function. The more obvious differences in beak form are also duplicated in the internal anatomy and functions of the oral cavity and alimentary canal. Although many species are quite adaptable, failure to appreciate a bird's normal feeding methods could lead to difficulties in prehension and an inadequate food intake. Parrots, for example, vary considerably in size and need seed which is applicable to their size. Lorikeets, although belonging to the

---

* 'Convalescent Diet'; (Pedigree Pet Foods).

psittacines and looking like small parrots, are adapted to eating fruit.

For most granivorous species the local pet shop can usually supply suitable seed foods and they may also be able to supply more specialized foods such as 'Sluis Universal' which is suitable for feeding insectivorous birds. Granivorous birds also require grit which needs to be the right size for a particular species. However, there is scientific evidence that some birds may be able to manage without grit.

Most raptorial birds can be maintained for quite long periods on the dead male chicks obtained from hatcheries. If one is constantly dealing with raptors a supply of hatchery chicks can be kept in a deep freeze. However, some raptors may not readily recognize and eat this food at first so it may be necessary to quarter the chick and expose the viscera. It may also be necessary to feed portions of the carcass by hand. If this is done, it is best to discard the head and any sharp parts of the skeleton. A normal healthy bird will deal with these but a weak bird may be injured by them. The pieces of meat can be offered with the fingers or, in the case of the more powerful bird of prey with forceps. The tips of these are best covered with tape to protect the points from damaging the orpharynx, and they must also be kept scrupulously clean. When feeding by mouth, if the sensitive vibrissae at the sides of the mouth, present in some species, are touched the bird will often grab at the food. If the mouth has to be opened by hand the upper beak or premaxilla can easily be raised which has the effect, through the rod like articulations of the palato-pterygoid and jugal bones connected to the quadrate bone, of depressing the lower beak or mandible.

Hatchery chicks are also suitable food for, and may be taken quite readily by, herons (Ardeidae), cormorants (Phalacrocoracidae), and birds of the crow family (Corvidae). If hatchery chicks are not readily available, small pieces of meat supplemented with vitamins and minerals and mixed with fur and feathers to provide roughage can be given. Always moisten these morsels of food before feeding. Combings of hair from any cat or dog will suffice as roughage in an emergency. As mentioned on pages 2 and 3 all raptors and in many other species of birds, regularly produce oral pellets. However, some parts of the skeleton of the prey are digested and are essential, particularly in young, growing raptors if metabolic bone disease is to be avoided. If hospitalized birds of prey do not produce pellets this usually means there is something wrong with the alimentary canal. Nevertheless, if there is insufficient roughage there is no scientific evidence that the production of pellets is essential to the normal function of the alimentary canal.

In the piscivorous species the provision of a fish diet is probably not essential to health. However, these birds will not often feed voluntarily unless the food offered looks like fish, and in some cases unless it is given in water and moves like a fish. Many types of birds only recognize food presented in a familiar form. Once over this difficulty they often thrive on an artifical diet.

Most of the gulls will feed readily on tinned pet food, but forced-feeding of this group of birds is difficult since food is stored in the lower oesophagus and easily regurgitated. Fulmars can eject an evil-smelling oil from the oesophagus a distance of 2—3 feet; vomiting in other species of birds is usually an indication of upper alimentary disease. When feeding gannets, care should be taken with the sharp edge of their beaks.

Physiotherapy

Many injured birds received into a veterinary practice will have trauma to muscle and tendons and to the nerve supply to these tissues. They may also be suffering from concussion. Any fracture present must first be treated; much can be done by intelligent nursing to restore the function of damaged soft tissue.

The nurse must always be aware that hospitalized birds are like human athletes who are out of regular training. The longer they are hospitalized the greater will be the deterioration in the cardiovascular and muscular systems due to disuse atrophy.

Faradism has been used to restore the function in a barn owl's leg Randell (L., 1980; personal communication), but this is unlikely to be available in most veterinary practices. Immersion of an injured limb in hot water at 114°F (45.5°C) and gentle flexion and extension of the joint as advised by Ratcliffe (J., 1982; personal communication) is simple and can often restore function.

McKeever (1979) recommends the use of a sling and neck brace supports for birds with neurological injuries when the bird cannot support its own weight or the head cannot be held up. The writer has successfully suspended a pigeon in a plastic bag for a total of three weeks whilst both fractured legs were allowed to heal, and has used this support in a Harris's Hawk (*Parabuteo unicinctus*) requiring simultaneous operations on both legs.

Once function has been restored to the muscles and other soft tissues these need to be strengthened and built up again. A bird will often do this if it is kept in a large cage or aviary but this can also be encouraged by daily exercising the patient. The bird can at first be held by the legs by hand (gloved if a raptor) and gently raised and lowered to stimulate wing flapping. Later exercise on a leash can be helpful. The leash can be attached to all types of birds by small soft leather straps or jesses as used by falconers, providing of course the legs of the species are stout enough for this purpose.

8 / Breeding Problems

Increasing demand and monetary value coupled with greater restrictions on supply because of nature conservation will result in more bird owners breeding from stock. The novice will try to replace his losses. The experienced breeder will want to breed for profit and hope to increase his output. Veterinary advice will be sought if these ambitions are to be achieved.

British birds and those from temperate climates breed during a few months of the summer when there is a maximum food supply and favourable weather. Some of the cage birds kept by aviculturists have evolved in tropical conditions but they have been bred in captivity for so long as to be almost domesticated. They are capable of breeding throughout the year and, if kept in outside aviaries, sometimes attempt to breed when the weather is most unsuitable. This can occur in parrots, exotic doves and small finches such as zebra and Bengalese.

Successful bird breeding needs luck, good management and some understanding of the natural history of the species. The breeder should have an empathy with his birds and sense their needs. The zebra finch breeds so easily that the veterinarian may even be asked how to stop them breeding. The solution is to remove the nest boxes and nesting materials or even to separate the sexes.

Failure to breed can be due to many causes. These can be catalogued under the following four headings: (i) failure to mate; (ii) inability to produce a normal fertile egg; (iii) failure of the fertile egg to hatch; (iv) failure to rear young.

Some reasons for failure to breed have a single cause but many are multifactorial with varying consequences dependent on the precedence of the different factors.

Failure to mate

A not uncommon reason being to have a pair of monomorphic birds of the same sex. Homosexuality sometimes occurs in birds. Two isolated male lovebirds may copulate and appear to mate normally. The only solution is to sex the birds.

CHAPTER 8

Sexing birds

This can be carried out by several methods. One is direct visual inspection of the cloacal anatomy, as used in poultry. Not usually practical in the smaller species but it is possible for an experienced operator to carry this out on mature specimens of some of the larger parrots. Two other possible methods of sexing birds are to examine either the chromosomal karyotype (from a blood sample) or to compare the relative concentrations of male and female hormones in the faeces. Both techniques require the help of a specialized laboratory and neither method has been well researched. Some breeders claim to be able to determine sex by measuring the width between the pelvic bones or by noting a slight difference in the lie of the feathering. Both measures are subjective and unreliable.

At present the most direct and reliable method is by surgical sexing. The technique has the added advantage that the conditions of the gonads can also be seen at the same time. The technique is described under laparoscopy in Chapter 2, pp. 27–33).

Stress and aggression

Two birds of opposite sex may not be compatible and dependent on the species, either sex can dominate the other. At worst this can lead to death of the submissive partner or at best infertility due to stress. Sometimes a change of partner, a larger aviary, or more feeding points or nest boxes may solve the problem. The latter is particularly important with falcons, weaver birds and whydahs. Persecution by other species in the same aviary will stop breeding. Some species are imcompatible and in some cases such as the small tropical doves, they will not tolerate another breeding pair of their own kind.

Occasionally a neurotic and aggressive bird will be encountered amongst a normal breeding group of budgerigars. This one bird can upset the whole flock.

Birds need to be reasonably tame and used to their keeper. Wild birds are reluctant to breed in captivity. It has been demonstrated by Burnham, Walton & Weaver (1983) that peregrine falcons taken from the wild breed less rapidly than those bred in captivity. Stress can be induced by excessive noise or any change in the birds' routine management. Observations of shy breeding pairs, such as falcons, can be carried out by a one-way glass window. Prowling predators, such as foxes, domestic cats and rodents around the aviary can disturb birds and prevent mating. Transportation can cause stress. After capture, foreign species are held by the dealer abroad, then transported by air. They usually undergo a period of quarantine before being sold to their final owners after possibly going through a series of traders. They may take a long time to become adjusted to their ultimate circumstances and then become ready to breed.

The breeder must realize that all birds are individuals in their behaviour, copulation and courtship, and allowances must be made for this. It may take 1 or 2 years for a breeding pair to become properly adjusted so that they copulate and produce fertile eggs.

One of a breeding pair may not be sexually mature. Many birds are mature in one year but some of the very large birds of prey may take several years, the macaws take 4 years and the psittacula parakeets, such as the Alexandrine and plum-headed take 3 years to reach maturity. Nevertheless, in most cases if a pair of birds have not bred after 3 years they are unlikely to do so.

Breeding birds should be in good physical condition, good examples of the species and not obviously suffering from any disease. They should not be obese. This is quite a common problem with captive and disabled raptors which are often overfed and underexercised. However, the bird must receive food in excess of its metabolic maintenance requirement. The cold weather of a late spring in temperate climates delays breeding in wild birds because they need more food for maintenance (Elkins, 1983). A sudden spell of mild weather stimulates song, courtship and pairing in wild birds and influences captive specimens as well. The increasing number of daylight hours has a major influence on sexual activity providing the above mentioned climatic and nutritional influences are favourable. Increasing the photo period in an aviary can help induce breeding. However, the irregular use of artificial lighting can have an adverse effect and therefore it is best to use a time switch.

Disease

Only after all the aforementioned factors have been taken into account should the clinician consider disease of the reproductive tracts of one or both breeding partners. General infectious disease is likely to exhibit other signs long before breeding is affected.

Toxic chemicals

Other remote influences are toxic chemicals, such as chlorinated hydrocarbons used in insecticides and the polychlorinated biphenyls widely used as industrial plasticizers and released when plastic materials are burned. It was thought initially that these compounds only caused thinning of the eggshell but it has been shown that they depress breeding by their influence on oestrogen levels (Peakall, 1970). Wood preserved with chemicals may be detrimental to parrots that chew it.

Inability to produce a normal fertile egg

Feeding

Breeding birds should be chosen from those individuals that will take a wide variety of foods and are not restricted in their feeding habits. In this way a deficiency of an essential element is less likely to occur. Some parrots for instance will eat sunflower seed and nothing else. Where possible home grown foods are better than those harvested abroad. Bird seeds grown in places like Morocco or parts of Australia are more likely to be cultivated on soils deficient in some mineral elements. If the viability of seed is in doubt sow some in a pot and let it sprout. If the green shoot looks normal the seed is probably all right.

Nesting sites

Birds seen to have mated may not have produced a fertile union because copulation took place on an insecure perch or one or both partners was inexperienced. Birds may not lay eggs in an aviary if there is not a suitably secure or sheltered nesting site or nesting material. It has been shown by Perrins (1979) that great tits and blue tits lay earlier in the season if they have warmer nesting boxes. Nest boxes for aviary birds are warmer if they are as small as practicable. As well as warmth, some hole nesting birds, such as parrots, need a sufficiently dark box to stimulate the hen to lay. This will not be achieved if there is a crack or warped joint in a wooden nest box. For these birds hollow logs make better nesting sites.

Egg laying

In all birds it is normal for the hen to look rather sick and suffer egg lethargy as egg laying becomes imminent. If the bird is disturbed whilst laying, she may drop the eggs anywhere in the aviary or may crack the shell. Egg eating is a habit formed by some birds which can turn into a vice copied by other birds in the aviary.

Infertile eggs are more liable to be laid by an old bird or one which has been allowed to raise too many broods in a season.

Candling

If access to the clutch can be gained without disturbing the hen, the eggs should be candled a few days after being laid. This enables one to decide if the egg is an infertile or 'clear' and to assess the condition of the egg shell, the air cell and the position of the embryo in the fertile egg. Candling can be carried out on thin-shelled eggs, such as those from parrots, using natural light. For others an artificial light source such as a 40 watt bulb can be used. For very thick-shelled eggs such as turkeys, some waterfowl and large raptors, an ultraviolet source is necessary. To avoid harm eggs should not be exposed to the candling light for more than a few seconds.

Artificial insemination

This has for many years been used routinely in poultry, and during the last decade the technique has been successfully developed for breeding raptors. The procedure described by Berry (1972), Boyd (1978), Bird et al. (1976), Grier et al. (1972), Grier (1973), Temple (1972) and Weaver (1983) has been evolved at a number of centres mainly in the U.S., but also in France (Wilkinson 1984).

The techniques of collection of semen in poultry and in raptors are essentially the same. They are to massage the lower part of the lumbo/sacral and abdominal regions in a rhythmic manner until a drop of semen is produced at the papilla in the cloaca. The papilla is gently held between thumb and forefinger. There is no technical reason why this technique could not be developed in other species of birds.

Boyd & Schwartz (1983) review the technique of semen collection used by a number of workers using a peregrine falcon imprinted onto its handler. An artificial pair bond is slowly formed between the handler and the gradually maturing young bird. This occurs after a long and intensive period of falconry training, including greeting the bird with a vocalization appropriate to its species and by food transfers. After this long period of socialization during which time a close physical and psychological relationship has been developed between bird and handler, the Tiercel will eventually copulate voluntarily with a specially designed hat worn by the handler. The hat carries a neoprene gutter around the brim which catches the semen. Using this technique semen can be collected several times a day over a period of a number of weeks.

To be successful the handler needs to understand and interpret correctly the courting displays that the bird makes to its 'artificial mate'. The whole process requires a lot of patience and complete dedication from the handler. For an excellent description of the technique the reader is referred to the publication by Boyd & Schwartz (1983).

Once collected the semen can be microscopically examined, or diluted with 50% ringers' solution before being used for inseminating the female. Avian semen is less liable to temperature shock than mammalian semen. Also in those species so far examined it is found to be less dense but the spermatozoa should all be the same size and mobile with no abnormalities of the head or tail. Semen should be collected early in the day before the birds are fed and after defaecation. It is then less likely to be contaminated with faeces and urates.

Insemination must be carried out at the correct time in the egg laying cycle. Weaver (1983) states this to be within six hours after the last egg was laid and favours insemination after each egg. However, in commerical poultry practice the birds are inseminated at 7—10 day intervals. Gilbert (1979) states that in those birds which have been examinined (mainly fowl-like birds and water fowl), the sperm is stored in the sperm host glands situated at the distal end of the oviduct. Fertilization, which takes place in the infundibulum at the proximal end of the oviduct, can occur several weeks after a single insemination. Gilbert thinks this is probably the case in all birds.

Failure of the fertile egg to hatch

This is probably the most common problem of all breeders and nearly always caused by a fault during incubation.

Development of the egg

During the first few days of incubation the respiratory needs of the developing embryo are supplied by simple diffusion of oxygen and carbon dioxide through the shell and its membranes. As the oxygen demands from the embryo increase, a network of capillary blood vessels form in the chorio allantoic membrane. Halfway through incubation this network lies under the whole of the inner shell membrane. Respiration is then taking place across the surface of the shell and oxygen is pumped round by the embryonic heart. Dunker (1977) states that at the end of incubation the embryo absorbs the amniotic fluid and the remainder of the albumen (the so called breakfast of the chicken). The amniotic cavity becomes aerated and air may penetrate the inner shell membrane. Respiratory movements become regular and serve to ventilate the lungs and air sac system before hatching. Unlike the respiratory system of the mammalian foetus, which undergoes further development after birth, the avian respiratory system is virtually complete and functioning at hatching.

The evolution of this method of development has enabled birds to create a constant-volume lung containing extremely thin-walled air capillaries. The minimum thickness barrier between the twin circulations of air and blood, together with a one-way flow of air, has made the avian lung the most efficient amongst the vertebrates. This has given birds the ability to reach high activity levels and to be able to fly at altitudes where levels of atmospheric oxygen are low. The developing egg with its delicate embryo and associated blood vessels is a fragile structure. Jerky movements, or vibration caused by nearby machinery, heavy lorries or children at play can all damage incubating eggs, particularly if held in an incubator.

The two most important environmental factors influencing incubation are temperature and relative humidity.

The influence of temperature

There is a narrow range of optimal temperatures for incubating eggs, which for poultry is 97°F–100.4°F and this has been found to be the same for falcons (Heck & Konke, 1983). The experienced bird will maintain the clutch within these limits. Incubating eggs can withstand some cooling, but not rises in temperature, which exceed those of the adult bird. Persistent low temperatures, due to cold weather prolong incubation and lead to small, weakly chicks with developmental abnormalities and unretracted yolk sacs. In wild birds, such as swifts and sea birds, where the incubation may have to be left for a period to enable the parent to forage, eggs have adapted to chilling without adverse effect (Elkin, 1983). Chilling of eggs with other birds can occur with a careless or inexperienced hen or from extreme weather with strong winds and rain. Draughty and damp nest boxes can lead to chilling. If birds are being bred inside, the optimum ambient temperature is about 60°F. Overheating of eggs, which could occur if they are in a faulty incubator or if they are exposed to the direct rays of the sun coming through a glass window, is lethal. If the embryo survives it is likely to be deformed.

The influence of humidity

Equally important to the survival of the embryo is the humidity around the egg. Most of the energy needs of embryonic development come from fat stored in the yolk. For every gram of fat metabolized an almost equal quantity of water is generated. If this water is not eliminated the embryonic tissues become waterlogged. Rahn et al. (1979) have pointed out that all eggs of whatever species need to lose as water about 15% of their initial weight at lay. This water loss needs to be evenly spread throughout the incubation period and leads to a gradual increase in size of the air cell at the blunt end of the egg. Failure of the egg to lose the correct amount of water leads to a tissue fluid imbalance. Insufficient loss of water vapour molecules through the shell is exactly paralleled by the low exchange rate of oxygen and carbon dioxide. The embryo becomes weak and may develop deformities. If the correct amount of water has been lost from the egg at the end of incubation, the shell is free to rotate around the embryo at hatching. If the egg is waterlogged the whole contents are too tight within the shell and this normal process cannot take place. For this reason dead-in-shell chicks are often found to be oedematous. Conversely, if the egg loses too much water the tissue becomes dehydrated and the air-cell is bigger than normal. In all cases of tissue fluid imbalance the chick lacks muscle tone and is unable to force its way out of the shell. In healthy and undisturbed female birds the desire to brood her clutch is very strong and she not only will make considerable efforts to maintain the eggs at both the correct temperature and humidity but will turn them regularly. Most species of birds develop a vascular brood patch over the breast, which transfers heat from the parent to the egg (King & McLelland, 1975). Frith (1959) has demonstrated that the incubator birds, the Megapodiidae are able to use the beak as a thermometer.

In an attempt to increase the humidity, some breeders will provide the nesting birds with damp nesting material. Fortunately this usually dries out before the eggs are laid so has little effect. Also some breeders will spray the eggs of a sitting hen with water to increase humidity. This is of doubtful benefit and may be harmful. The bird is best left to control the situation instinctively. Rahn *et al.* (1979) has shown that the relative humidity of the nest of most wild birds is kept at about 45%, which is about right for the eggs to lose the requisite amount of water.

Incubators

If eggs are incubated artifiically correct hatching conditions will have to be duplicated. Management of the incubator, even to the room in which it is kept will have to be meticulous. Temperature and relative humidity must be strictly controlled. Incubators are best kept in a room at a temperature of 70°F–80°F and the relative humidity should be kept low—no more than 50%. For safety, incubators should be controlled by double thermostats and any draughts or hot spots within the incubator should be identified. The eggs will need to be rotated eight times a day through 45° in alternate directions. Hygiene must be faultless and fumigation using a mixture of potassium permanganate (0.4 g) and formalin (0.8 cc of 37.5%) must be carried out at the end of the hatching season. The eggs must be weighed regularly to make sure the weight loss is correct. The weight can be checked against a graph indicating predicted weight loss. Considering that so few breeders follow these guide-lines it is surprising that any normal chicks are ever hatched.

Influence of the egg shell

Apart from the relative humidity of the microclimate around the egg, the most important factor controlling water loss is the egg shell. The exchange of water vapour, oxygen and carbon dioxide takes place through well-defined shell pores. The pattern and complexity of these channels varies with species. They are more complex in the larger species with thicker shells. Ar & Rahn (1977) have shown that in eggs that are of comparable weight and egg shell thickness the pore size is inversely proportional to the incubation period. Any factor that effects shell quality and shell thickness will have an effect on the porosity of the shell. This will affect gaseous exchange and egg weight loss during incubation. Abnormal shell may be caused by a variety of factors. There may be disease of the oviduct due to micro-organisms such as *E. coli* and *Mycoplasma*. The reasons may be genetic or due to the age of the hen. A dietary calcium/phosphorous imbalance (which should be calcium 1–5 parts to phosphorus 1 part) may result in soft-shelled eggs but is much more liable to result in cessation of egg laying. Soluble grit always must be available for herbivorous birds. There may be a deficiency of zinc, manganese or Vitamin D_3. Unlike mammals, birds are unable to metabolize Vitamin D_2. Use of sulphonamides and excessive use of antibiotics can affect shell quality. The chlorinated hydrocarbon DDT, its metabolyte DDE and dieldrin, as well as the polychlorinated biphenyls have been a notorious cause of thin-shelled eggs, not only in wild raptors but in many other birds such as pelicans and cormorants at the top of the food chain (Peakall, 1970). This cause is unlikely in captive birds unless insecticides have been used in an aviary to control insects, but this must always be taken into account. Shell quality can also be affected if the bird is stressed whilst the shell is being formed in the shell gland. Some birds such as parrots normally lay thin-shelled eggs which may be related to the more humid environment of a hole-nesting bird. Thin-shelled eggs tend to be laid in very hot weather. Hyperventilation by the bird to overcome hyperthermia leads to respiratory alkalosis. This results in a lowering of the partial pressure of carbon dioxide in the blood with the result that less calcium ions are available to the cells of the shell gland. The cause of 50% of deaths in shell embryos takes place in the last few days of incubation and is due to adverse temperature and humidity during incubation.

Hatching

At the end of incubation, which varies with species, the egg hatches. Incubation times are given in Appendix 2. A few hours prior to hatching the embryo, using its egg tooth, pierces the internal shell membrane and starts to inhale from the enlarged air cell—a process known as internal pipping and chicks may start calling to each other at this time. Next a small crack indicating external pipping appears in the shell. The area around the crack starts to break up and eventually a flap with a sizeable hole develops.

The whole process is gradual, leading to the progressive functioning of the chick's respiratory and cardiovascular systems. Simultaneously, the yolk sac starts to retract into the chick and the blood vessels of the chorioallantois begin shutting down. From the start of external pipping to the emergence of the chick may take up to 24 hours. A weak chick will take longer. If the chick is taking too long to hatch there is a great temptation on the part of the anxious breeder to help it out of the shell—this is a mistake. There is a grave danger that the respiratory system may not be ready, the yolk sac may not be retracted and the chorioallantoic vessels may not be completely shut down. These vessels easily tear and a fatal haemorrhage can result. It is better to leave the chick at least 48 hours from the first sign of pipping or hearing the chick chirp and only then, if necessary, carefully extract it. The yolk sac may require ligating. Once the shell is open, fluid is lost more rapidly and prolonged hatching may lead to a dehydrated chick which will benefit from a little subcutanous sterile saline.

Infection of the egg

The chick embryo has long been the laboratory tool of the microbiologist. The avian embryo has no effective immunological defence mechanism, although passive immunity is acquired from the hen via the yolk. However, the antibodies probably do not pass into the embryonic circulation until about half-way through incubation. Before this, the egg is at greatest risk. Approximately 25% of dead in shell chicks die in the early stages of incubation due to infection. Infertile eggs can become infected and act as a focus for pathogenic organisms. Some breeders are in the habit of leaving unhatched eggs in the nest to give support to the chicks. It should not be forgotten that in some species such as parrots, owls and other raptors the eggs do not hatch out on the same day. There may be several days age between each chick. In passerines and many other birds, although the eggs do not hatch simultaneously there is very little interval between hatching. The egg can become infected any time from the start of its formation in the oviduct. However, the most common cause of infection is from dirty nest boxes or unhygienic incubators. All dead in shell eggs should be cultured for bacteria and fungi (p. 24). Cultures should be taken from the yolk sac, the albumen and the embryo's liver. The results of these cultures and a post-mortem examination on the embryo may give some indicaton as to how and when the egg was infected. The dead chick should be examined for any developmental abnormalities and its age should be estimated from the size relative to the egg. If pathogenic organisms are isolated, then an assessment of the whole nesting area or incubator together with bacteriological sampling needs to be made.

In summary the veterinarian investigating failure of the eggs to hatch needs to differentiate between the following common problems: Eggs that are infertile, those that are waterlogged or dehydrated and those that are infected. The investigation will also need to take into account other less common causes such as the age, nutrition and disease status of the hen and if the eggs have been handled and stored carelessly before incubation.

For more information the reader is referred to standard text books such as *Poultry Diseases* edited by R.F. Gordon.

Failure to rear the young

As well as deserting eggs, birds will sometimes abandon the chicks and cease to feed them at any stage of brooding. This may be caused by stress or it may be genetic or neurotic in origin. If a bird rears one year but not the next then stress as described in pp. 180–181 is the most likely cause. Similar to the situation in mammals, some birds will attack the chicks.

Fostering

If the survivors are rescued they will have to be reared artificially or by foster parents. These can readily be found from amongst such birds as zebra or Bengalese finches, redrump parrots, budgerigars, or, in the case of raptors, other falcons. Perrins (1979) found that wild blue tits will feed the young of blackbirds or treecreepers and wrens will feed coaltits. Fostering may result in the young bird becoming imprinted onto the species of the foster parents and may result in pairing difficulties when the birds reach sexual maturity and come to breed. This has not been demonstrated in wild birds. There is an increasing tendency for aviculturists to take the first clutch of eggs in an effort to encourage further laying by the hen. The first group of eggs is then incubated artificially. This may increase productivity but it is not a practice to be encouraged unless preformed by trained biologists.

The needs of birds feeding young

All breeding birds should have access to a shallow pan of water. This enables them not only to bathe but to take water, held in the breast feathers, to the chicks or eggs if necessary. Also, birds feeding young may have increased fluid requirements. Pigeons produce crop milk during the early part of brooding and there is increased flow of saliva in parrots rearing young. Smith (1982) suggests that this may have an effect on the activity of plant enzymes when the seed is held for some hours in the crop of the adult bird. This may increase the nutritive value of the food. Smith has shown that such regurgitated seed has a higher nutritive value than that fed to the adult bird. This worker also observes that the primitive bird, the hoatzin, may carry out fermentation in its crop similar to that taking place in the rumen of a cow. Baker (J.R., 1981; personal communication) notes that protozoa are normal inhabitants of the crop in the budgerigar.

Most of the seed-eating birds need to feed their young on animal protein, such as caterpillars and larvae of other insects. Mealworms and other live food should be provided by the aviculturist during this period. If birds such as parrots are fed too much green food or fruit, their droppings become very moist. This can lead to a damp, unhygienic nest with flies and maggots that will attack the chicks. Many wild birds go to considerable trouble to keep the nest clean either carrying away debris or trampling it into the dry material at the bottom of the nest. Passerines remove faecal sacs from the young and often, egg shells and dead chicks are removed from the nest by many species of birds. Young raptors instinctively defecate over the side of the nest or if ground nesters wander away from the nest to defecate.

The progress of growing chicks

Properly fed young should gain regularly in weight. A competent bird breeder whose birds are adjusted to him should be able to examine and weigh the chicks regularly. Some aviculturists do examine the chicks but few seem to weigh and record the progress of the chicks. If the weather is cold there may be some temporary loss of weight. Occasionally a chick may develop splayed legs, a condition seen in both raptors and psittacines. This usually is due to a chick being on an unsuitable, slippery surface during growth. If left untreated this can result in permanent damage. The condition can be treated using a figure-of-eight suture round the legs for about a week or putting the chick in a cup or small bowl which tends to push the legs under the body. The handling of parrot and falcon nestlings does not disturb them but if young passerines are handled 3–4 days prior to the time when they are due to leave the nest they may erupt and fledge prematurely.

During the first 10 days of brooding, the chicks are poikilothermic gradually becoming homoiothermic (Elkins, 1983). The adult birds will brood them continuously. During this period the feathers of altricial chicks begin to grow. The rate of growth varies among individual chicks. At the end of this period when the adults begin to spend less time keeping their brood warm, the least-feathered chicks are at greatest risk. The initial feather cover is not a very efficient heat insulator. Many young chicks die of chilling at this time. The chilled youngster becomes torpid, fails to beg for food and dies of starvation. Nest boxes that are too large, poorly insulated, damp or with only one or two chicks can become quite cold. The larger the number of fledglings in a nest, the greater the body mass and the smaller the ratio of surface area to body volume. Even the totally feathered and active praecocial chicks of water-fowl sustain considerable losses if there are adverse weather conditions during the first weeks of life.

Artificial rearing

If chicks are reared artificially in a hatcher, the temperature will need to be reduced progressively during the growing period. As the feathers grow the breeder should take note from their behaviour if the chicks are too hot or too cold and adjust the temperature accordingly. A hot chick will lie with wings and legs stretched out and will keep away from other chicks. Cold chicks huddle together or, if by themselves, wander around their enclosure. In both cases they tend to make a lot of noise. The breeder should try to access if a chick's crop and stomach are being filled properly. This may either be felt or seen through the semi-transparent skin of the neck and abdomen.

In conclusion it should be stressed that the three most common causes of death in nestlings are hypothermia, starvation and infection. Infanticide is not uncommon and such factors as vitamin and mineral deficiencies and chemical toxins occasionally increase mortality.

9 / The Release of Casualty Wild Birds

Factors that affect survival

Considerable interest has been shown and much has been written during the last two decades about the rehabilitation of injured wild raptors. This knowledge has been developed particularly in the United States with the foundation of such organisations as the 'Raptor Research and Rehabilitation Program' based at the University of Minnesota. Concern about raptors is important, since this group of birds is at the greatest risk from extinction. Raptors are often in direct conflict with man and being at the top of the food chain they are most liable to the cumulative effects of the toxic agricultural chemicals. However, the veterinarian in practice is often presented with other groups of sick and injured wild birds, some of which he will want to release. The factors that must be taken into account when birds other than raptors are released vary tremendously. Comparatively little has been written about this aspect of the problem and this chapter is an attempt to examine the task as it affects all species of birds.

As will be seen in the following pages, the release of wild birds is something which should not be undertaken lightly. It not only requires skill as an avian clinician but also knowledge of the bird's natural history. Cooper (1979) has pointed out that in the United Kingdom under the Abandonment of Animals Act 1960, 'the indiscriminate release of wild bird casualties without careful consideration of their chance of survival in the wild could amount to an offence.' On the other hand, any person who keeps any wild bird that could be released is guilty of an offence under the Wildlife and Country Act 1981.

The factors can be broadly divided into two areas which are to some extent inter-related. Firstly, there is the bird's physical and mental fitness to cope with its environment. Secondly, the habitat into which it is released. This is constantly changing and unless a bird is to be released where it was found within a few days of injury, there are many aspects that must be considered. A bird that is in the wrong environment and not completely fit will not only be unable to feed itself properly but will soon be spotted by a predator even if that bird looks normal to the casual observer.

The assessment of physical fitness

Whilst it is generally true that a bird needs to be anatomically perfect and 100% fit before release it is not entirely necessary. How much disability a bird can adapt to will depend a great deal on its normal patterns of behaviour.

Skeletal damage

A healed fracture of the humerus or the ulna may not be in perfect alignment and there may have been some shortening of the bone but many birds will still be able to fly. There are a number of recorded instances where birds have been found surviving with malaligned, healed fractures (Olney, 1958/1979; Tiemier, 1941; Hurrel, 1968). The author has seen several cases in raptors where the fracture had not healed perfectly but where the bird had mated and successfully reared young. This indicates that the bird was hunting effectively enough not only to survive but also to catch enough food for its young. Quite obviously these birds had learned to compensate for the disparity between the normal and abnormal wing.

What is much more important for the bird to be able to fly efficiently is movement in its wing joints. Even here some slight loss in the range of movement may be tolerable and a bird may learn to adapt. A short-winged hawk such as a sparrowhawk or goshawk may be able to cope with the loss of 10% range of movement in its carpal joints. These creatures are birds of fast forward flight and a high wing loading and a high tail-surface-to-wing-surface ratio. Once airborne the momentum of the bird helps to keep it in the air. Steering and braking depend on the tail. Ducks and pigeons are also birds with short, broad wings and fast forward flight.

On the other hand a bird such as a barn owl or harrier has quite a different mode of flight. The wing loading is lower, particularly in the owl and full mobility of the carpal joints is essential for the birds manoeuverability. These birds need the maximum lift on their wings to hunt—slowly quartering the ground and in the case of the owl pivoting in the air. A barn owl with an ankylosed elbow joint was seen to be able to ascend and to glide, but once it tried to turn it completely collapsed.

Large, soaring birds of prey need complete mobility in the digital and carpal joints. The muscles of this area are well developed. The large emarginated primary feathers are splayed out and act like slots in an aeroplane wing to reduce turbulence and increase lift. The distance between the slots is constantly being adjusted by the bird. In the soaring gull mobility of the carpal joint is not so important so long as it can extend the wing completely.

The kestrel, which spends much time hovering to catch its prey, probably needs complete mobility in all the wing joints. Hovering requires more energy than fast forward flight so that it is possible that the kestrel needs to be a more efficient predator than the sparrow-hawk.

Soft tissue damage to the locomotory system

Some muscles may have been so badly damaged as to be permanently atrophied. The propatagial membrane is often injured in collisions and if scar tissue results, extension of the wing may be severely affected. The author has seen cases where the leading edge of the wing is placed more than one inch posteriorly to the body, than that on the normal side. In these cases flight is affected. In a less severly disabled case the bird may be able to fly but lift on the affected side is reduced because of a reduction in effective wing area. The bird may compensate by trimming the normal wing so that both wings are equal in area and also by flying a bit faster (Fig. 9.1). Lift on an aerofoil, be it a bird's wing or an aeroplane, is not only proportional to the effective wing area but is proportional to the square of the relative wind speed. The author has seen a case of damage to the propatagial membrane in a Harris' hawk where the bird was able to fly but constantly veered off to the left. Quite obviously this bird would not have survived in the wild.

Small birds such as wrens, blackbirds and tits which live in dense woodland cover and do not normally fly great distances may survive with wings which are not quite normal. Providing the distance between perching positions is not too great these birds will adapt. However, if they are released in a more open habitat where the distance between trees and bushes is greater they will be at a disadvantage. They are unable to glide properly like the short wing hawk and ducks mentioned earlier—although they have short broad wings, the frontal body surface area in relation to their body mass is high (i.e. the profile drag is high) and they don't have sufficient momentum to carry them forward. Small birds such as the wren, the robin and the starling need to be able to manoeuvre accurately to be

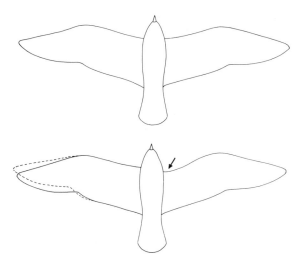

Fig. 9.1 (a) This shows the position of the wings in a normal bird.
(b) This shows how the bird trims the wing on the uninjured side by slight flexion
to balance the abnormal wing. The arrow indicates the position of the scarred and
displaced propatagial membrane. To get the same amount of lift, (b) flies slightly
faster than (a).

able to get into and out of their hole nesting sites. However, small
birds do have an advantage over the large birds. They can sustain a
proportionately larger amount of permanent damage to their main
flight muscles than can large birds. This is because the power margin,
(the energy available from the muscles required to lift the bird into the
air and keep it airborne, beyond the minimum power required for this
activity) is much greater in small birds. In a bird the size of a swan or
large vulture which cannot jump into the air but has to have some
distance or a strong head wind to get up relative air speed, the power
margin is low. The bird, in fact, only just makes it. Very little damage
needs to occur to the soft tissue of these large birds and they won't fly
again.

No two species of birds have the same flight pattern and probably
no two individual birds fly in exactly the same manner, just as no two
people walk exactly the same.

How a partially disabled bird learns to fly again will depend on the
particular disability and on behaviour pattern of that species. So that a
considered judgement can be made on these matters it is important
that the clinician carries out a thorough physical examination of his

patient before release is considered. This should preferably include the use of X-rays, the examination of the mobility of all wing joints together with the extensibility of the wings. This should be carried out systematically even if no fractures of the wings occured. This examination can only be done properly if the bird is relaxed under anaesthesia. One cannot properly compare the mobility of the joints in each wing in the conscious bird and it is easy to miss a slightly damaged propatagial membrane.

A bird may look normal when it is alert and perching under observation. Once the observer has disappeared the bird relaxes and both wings may not be held symmetrically.

A bird may feel round and in good condition, its weight may be normal for the species and time of year, but the weight may just be fat. If a bird has been in captivity for sometime the ratio of fat to muscle may be too high. Nevertheless some fat must be present as an energy reserve.

Testing flying ability

Having considered all the above factors there is only really one way to assess a bird's flying ability and that is to see it fly. To a limited extent this may be possible in a large aviary. The larger the aviary in relation to the size of the bird the better. Much information can be gained by watching the bird fly in a garage or barn. It may be possible to give the bird daily exercise with these facilities to build up the bird's fitness. Ideally the enclosure needs to be as high and as long as possible. The bird can then practice gaining in height as well as propelling itself forward.

Falconers have developed methods of flying birds on a leash. This is light in weight and the bird is allowed to trail up to 100 metres which enables it to be controlled. A large open space is essential with no obstructions and no distractions for the bird. If possible it is best to fly the bird uphill and with the wind behind it. This makes flying much harder work and gives a better assessment of how well the bird can fly. This technique is applicable to other types of birds besides raptors. Such birds as pigeons, ducks and gulls, with strong legs are suitable but the method cannot be used in those species with long legs such as herons or waders or any bird with delicate legs.

The method only tests the ability to fly in a straight line, it does not show if the bird can gain height or show how it can manoeuvre. These skills really can be tested only in a large, confined space. If after allowing the bird to fly for a short distance it is dyspnoeic for more than a few seconds it is not fit to release. A normal bird should be able to fly long distances without getting into respiratory distress.

Loss of feathers and damage to the plumage

Before releasing, the plumage must be in good order. Not only must most of the main flight feathers be present but the thermal, insulating properties of the covert feathers must be effective. Many birds can fly with a few feathers missing—they often do so when moulting but the loss of these flight feathers must not form large gaps in the aerofoil section of the wing. Large birds have an irregular pattern of moulting because they cannot afford to lose too many feathers to remain airborne. Waterfowl become flightless during moulting. Lorenz (1965) cut off different sections of the remiges in pigeons to see what effect this had on flight. When most of the primary flight feathers had been removed the bird could still fly in level flight but could not ascend. If the secondary flight feathers were progressively removed level flight was affected, although height could be gained.

Falconers use the technique of imping to replace a damaged feather with one that has been moulted or one that has been obtained from a casualty bird. The feather does not have to be from the same species, although the feather must not only be approximately the right size but must be of the same texture. The flight feathers of chickens and pheasants are harder than those of other birds. The shape must be right. In many large birds, particularly the raptors, the outer primaries are emarginated, the vane on one side of the shaft is very much narrower for part of its length.

The technique of imping is applicable to birds other than raptors. The shaft of the broken feather is cut below the damaged area and the shaft of the new feather is cut so that the upper part replaces the faulty section. The two halves are joined together with a peg made of bamboo, a needle, or the quill of another feather of suitable diameter. Any substances can be used so long as it is the right diameter to be inserted into the ends of the two cut shafts and is strong enough. The whole is held in place with glue.

A new feather can be stimulated to grow by gently pulling out the stump of the old feather. However, growth of the new feather takes time.

The loss of tail feathers is more important in some birds than others. Many can fly without the tail but birds such as sparrow-hawks, hen harriers, magpies, gulls and kites cannot steer properly. The kestrel, the buzzard and the tern cannot hover. The large eagles and the owls can probably manage better than most but the precision of flying will be affected.

Damage to the legs

The full functioning of both legs is probably not so important as that of the wings. Fishing line can eventually lead to gangrene and loss of part of the leg. Some birds lose toes through frost bite. All these birds can and do survive. Some rotation of the tibio tarsus after healing is also quite tolerable. The legs are more important to a raptor but there are reports of these birds hunting and surviving with only one leg functional. Nevertheless the chances of a heavy bird such as a buzzard developing bumble-foot infection are greatly increased if it is constantly standing on one foot. Species such as the heron are severly handicapped in their methods of hunting with one leg.

Damage to the eyes

The loss of an eye might be thought to be a severe handicap which would affect the judgment of distance but this is not always so. Birds can manage with one eye and are able to judge distance sufficiently accurately to be able to land with precision on a branch. Brown (1978) in a personal communication, records such a case in a female crowned eagle (*Stephandaetus coronatus*). This bird survived at least two years with what appeared to be a cataract in one eye. However, Brown notes that the breeding success of this bird was reduced after it developed disease of the eye. It was then probably not a completely efficient predator.

In the peregrine falcon two perfect eyes would be essential. These birds may start their attack on a victim anything from 500 metres to 4.5 kilometres away from the target (Brown 1976).

The author has known two owls and a buzzard in which loss of an eye occured and the birds were able to survive.

In the prey species the bird may survive but its chances of eluding a predator would be reduced.

The importance of good hearing

In birds such as owls or harriers which have sustained damage to the head, the clinician should consider if the hearing of the bird is likely to be affected. Both these groups quarter the ground they are hunting with a slow methodical flight, using their facial discs to pick up the slightest sound. Hearing in these birds is more important than sight. Hearing may be important to some invertebrate feeders. Certainly the thrushes locate earthworms by listening.

Mental health

When considering if a bird's behaviour pattern will enable survival in environment, casualties can be divided into two fundamentally different groups.

Firstly there are those birds that were mature when first caught. These birds have learned to find food for themselves. Provided they still retain their natural fear of man and his domestic animals they pose little problem. Granted if this group are not kept in captivity for more than about 14 days they soon resort to their old habits. If they are released into the exact location where they were found then they know the local geography and where the likely food sources are situated. This group usually survives very well.

If a bird has been captive for several months before it is released it may take a little time to get back to its normal routine. Apart from being out of the habit of continually having to search for food, the bird's food supply will have changed. Summer has changed to autumn or winter. Abundant supplies of insects and vegetable food have changed. Many small birds have migrated and the countryside which yielded a plentiful supply of easily caught young animals for the predator has disappeared. The released casualty will need support feeding from a familiar source whilst it is learning to adapt to the changed situation.

The group of birds that pose the greatest problem for release are the young which may have been captured at some stage of their development. These birds, which have never lived freely, not only may have to be taught to search for food but may develop undesirable characteristics during their nursing period.

The altrical nestings, which include the raptors, are fed by the parents not only during the time they are in the nest but also for a period after they have left the nest. During this post-fledging period the young bird is not only developing the skills of flying but also, in the case of predators, is learning to hunt and catch prey successfully. Foraging for food in the prey species may also be partly learned by watching parents and also by natural curiosity and investigating all strange objects. Jones,(C.S., 1984; personal communication) has noted that the rate at which young tawny owls learn to fly and pounce accurately on a moving prey, varies between individuals. Some birds may never become quite so good as others.

Young raptors can be taught to hunt by traditional falconry methods using feeding from the fist, feeding to the lure and 'waiting on' etc. The reader is referred to standard texts on falconry such as Mavrogordato's *A Hawk for the Bush* (1960) and Woodford's *A Manual of Falconry* (1960). A raptor will learn to hunt if it is confined to a barn where there are live mice or rats or if it is in an aviary where small mammals and birds can get through the mesh of the netting but through which the predator cannot escape. To feed live animals to a bird of prey is illegal in the United Kingdom under the Protection of Animals Act 1911–1964.

In the precocial species such as pheasants, plovers and waterfowl, where the young hatch fully feathered, feeding behaviour is almost entirely instinctive but these birds do need to be exposed to their normal habitat during the developing period so that they will learn to investigate all types of potential food items such as invertebrates.

Imprinting

This phenomenon, first demonstrated by Lorenz in geese (1935 and 1937), is seen in all species and has far reaching implications. As the young bird matures its mental awareness of its environment becomes more acute. The bird recognizes not only its parents which feed it but also its siblings, nest site and food. These images become fixed in that part of the nervous system controlling behaviour. Alter any of these normal contacts in the developing young bird's environment and problems of behaviour occur. The bird fails to recognize or has difficulty in recognizing its own species when it reaches maturity. If raptors are not presented with a variety of their normal prey species they may never learn to hunt properly. All birds have great difficulty recognizing food items with which they are not familiar although they may be quite suitable as food. Feed a developing raptor entirely on hatchery chicks and it becomes imprinted on them.

Birds often return to the same nest, possibly because the surrounding environment is imprinted on them.

Young fledglings reared and hand fed by humans become imprinted on the handler. They continue to beg for food and can become totally dependent on their human benefactor. These birds may never pair and mate with their own species because they do not recognize them. They may in fact form a sexual pair bond with their human rescuer. When such birds are released they may attack unsuspecting humans in the belief that these persons are a natural food source or that they are a natural mate. McKeever (1979) thought that human imprinted owls released into the wild could be dangerous. In the more rapacious species injury to humans could be severe. Each year newspaper reports appear, usually towards the end of the summer or in the autumn, of a demented owl which has attacked someone. These may be imprinted birds released by well meaning but ignorant do-gooders.

The critical period of socialization takes place in different groups at different stages of development. In the altrical nesting it is generally later and longer than in the precocial chick. The rigidity of imprinting probably also varies with the species.

Some authorities believe that imprinting can never be reversed. Certainly it is difficult and may take years. For the biologist intent on breeding his rare captive raptor this may be practical. For the clinician who wants to release a wild bird after treatment, imprinting can produce insuperable problems.

Reversion to juvenile behaviour by an injured bird can sometimes occur (Lack, 1975) and the author has noticed this in an injured parrot which had lost its upper beak. Reverted mature birds open their mouths and at the same time carry out slight fluttering movements of the wings begging for food.

If a young bird is reared, by a well meaning person, in complete isolation in an attempt to stop imprinting onto its human contact, it becomes completely neurotic. It is hypersensitive, frightened of its own shadow and fears all living things—a phenomenon not confined to birds. These birds are excessively aggressive and frightened of their surroundings. A good discussion of abnormal and maladaptive behaviour which is important to the releaser of wild birds is given by Jones (1980).

The environment where the bird is to be released

Taking this into account is an equally important part of the problem of releasing wild birds. The summer period in temperate climates is a time of plentiful food supply. Birds that are physically and mentally fit should have no difficulty in finding sufficient food. However, at the beginning of the summer period, there is often intense competition amongst conspecifics for breeding territory. This biological phenomenon is an attempt on the part of the breeding birds to map out and familiarize themselves with a secure food supply on which to rear their young. An outsider of the same species or even a competitive species released into this territory comes under considerable stress through constant attack and harassment. This is no good for a bird which is trying to rehabilitate itself into the environment.

It would be wiser to pick an area in which to release where the food supply is plentiful but where the number of suitable nesting sites is restricted (Newton, 1979).

As the summer period advances the ground cover in a wood increases and makes it harder for the tawny owl to hunt for its food. But this is an easier time for the prey species including many small birds, food is abundant and it is easier to hide from the predator. As autumn turns to winter, the ground cover is much less dense giving fewer refuges for the prey and the balance shifts in favour of the owl. These constantly changing circumstances favouring first one group of birds, then another takes place to some extent in all types of habitat. They should always be considered instead of simply releasing the bird. Many birds are migratory, being only in the United Kingdom for a relatively short period during the summer to breed. By the time they are fit for release the food supply of insectivores such as swifts, swallows and warblers may have gone.

The short-eared owl and the hen harrier breed on the upland moor during the summer but migrate locally to the estuaries and lowlands during the winter.

Before any bird is released into a habitat it is essential that the releaser makes sure that an adequate food supply is available. The habitat may look right—it does not necessarily mean that the food, for instance the prey species, are present. It is therefore important that to be successful in releasing casualty birds, the veterinarian should either be a competent naturalist or have the cooperation of such a person. The County Naturalists Trusts or the RSPB local groups can be contacted for help. The correct assessment of the complex interactions of the bird and the environment requires a wealth of knowledge of natural history and some practical skill as a field naturalist.

The weather

This is another important and complicated consideration. Prolonged heavy rain can severly restrict the feeding of many species—from the aerial insectivores to the hovering species such as the kestrel. For the barn owl and harrier rain reduces the acuity of hearing. Sea shore waders, and small birds feeding in dense foliage such as the wren, are less affected.

Just after heavy rain there are often many invertebrates, particularly earthworms, near the surface. In dry weather, particularly if prolonged, the invertebrates migrate deeper into the soil. In wetland areas during the drought soil increases in salinity so that fewer invertebrates are available.

Cold weather is important especially if the ground is frozen. Under these conditions the balance between the energy intake of the bird and its energy losses in searching for food and maintaining body temperature may be critical. It is therefore important that the bird has adequate fat reserves before release. Even the barn owl probably only stores sufficient fat reserves to last 3 days. In small birds the energy reserve is much less. Unless the cold weather is very severe the sea shore and estuarine mud is unlikely to freeze as it is periodically warmed by the tide. However, the invertebrates travel deeper in cold weather so that the species feeding near the surface with short beaks are disadvantaged. The wind chill factor with high wind in low temperature can lead to the loss of a lot of body heat. Prolonged frost can have disastrous effects on woodland birds feeding on the pupae and eggs of insects secreted in the bark of trees.

Wind and cold have less effect near the ground and on the leeward side of a wood but are important in the woodland clearings.

High wind churns up large expanses of water including the sea. This stirs up bottom mud making feeding for diving species difficult. A rough sea pounding a rocky shore constantly disturbs the purple sandpiper and the turnstone so that they can spend less time feeding. The subject of weather and bird behaviour is very well covered by Elkins (1983).

Because of all these factors it is wise to consider the weather forecast the next few days before releasing a bird.

Other factors to be considered before releasing casualty birds

Birds should be released at first light or as early in the day as possible. This gives them the maximum feeding period before darkness and gives them as much time as possible to orientate themselves.

A prey species such as a small tit, a plover or a starling may stand a better chance of survival if it is released near a flock of the same or similar species. Even here there is often a pecking order and the bird will be under some stress until it is accepted.

It is unwise to release birds near a busy main road. Many owls and other species such as crows are attracted to the small vertebrate casualties killed on the road and themselves become injured or killed. Even small birds such as wrens, robins and thrushes tend to fly low over road-ways and become casualties. Some birds of prey such as the buzzard, the little owl and the short-eared owl use telegraph poles or fence posts alongside the road as perches to watch for prey.

When releasing raptors onto farmland or near large estates it is better to have the permission and cooperation of the occupier of the land and his staff.

Releasing a sparrowhawk near an industrial estate or where there is a large complex of buildings would be unwise. These birds often chase prey into a building and then become trapped. The netting of a fruit farm is a similar hazard. Barbed wire fences across open farmland are a particular hazard to barn owls. Swans need a large expanse of water with no overhead wires.

The techniques of release

As stated earlier when a bird is building up its strength and initially learning to fly, or convalescing after injury it can be kept in an aviary or other suitable enclosure. If this is situated in a suitable area for release, when the time comes to let the bird go, the netting on the top of the aviary can be rolled back quietly. This method has several advantages. The bird has become familiar with the surrounding territory. It can go back to the aviary as a temporary refuge and this can also be a source of support food whilst the bird learns to forage for itself.

A method that has been used successfully to release falcons is to use a 'hack box'. This is basically the same principle as the aviary method except that it is portable. The box is really a small cage, the size dependent on the species. For falcons it should be about $6' \times 4' \times 4'$. The box is transported to the site chosen for release and left containing the bird on site for 7–10 days. The box needs to be well protected from predators. During this time the bird is fed from behind a screen or using a chute so that the handler cannot be seen. The principle is to try and break the feeding bond and give the bird time to familiarize itself with the surrounding area. At the end of the habituation period the cage is opened but feeding continues for long enough to make sure the bird is foraging for itself. Support feeding may need to be gradually reduced to encourage normal hunting.

Both of the above methods are suitable for most types of birds but may need some modification. Raptors can be released after using standard hacking back techniques. After training they can be tethered to a 'hack board'. This is a wooden platform which acts like an artificial nest site. The bird is tethered for several days, during which time it is fed and gets to know the neighbouring territory, and then is released. Some falconers suggest carrying the bird on the fist around the area surrounding the hack board for several days prior to release. This helps familiarize the bird with its territory. Regular feeding on the hack board continues and is gradually reduced to encourage hunting.

Survival of all species depends not only on the physical and mental well-being of the bird but also on it having an intimate knowledge of its local environment so that it can find food and shelter.

Conclusion

It can be appreciated that the problem of releasing the casualty after treatment is complex. The work can be time consuming and frustrating, because a bird may die at any stage in the rehabilitation process (Appendix 10). However, it is important that veterinary surgeons should be involved in this work and in cooperation with other natural scientists should record their experiences and observations so that others can make use of these records and build on them. The veterinarians expertise and skill used in this way can help to make some positive contribution to conservation. The techniques worked out on common species can be used on the rarer birds. Today's common bird may become tomorrow's rarity or even become extinct, like the passenger pigeon, which was so numerous in North America during the early part of the 19th century, that during migration flocks containing two billion birds would darken the sky. As H.R.H. Prince Philip has stated, 'It is absolutely inevitable that a very large number of species are going to become extinct in spite of our best efforts'. The Prince warned that in not protecting wildlife our own days will be numbered—'for we simply cannot survive without the other living species that co-exist with us on this planet'.

Appendices

1/Weights of birds most likely to be seen in general practice

The birds marked with an asterisk (*) are the species mentioned in the text.

Common name	Scientific name	Weight range in grams
Order: Psittaciformes		
Lesser Sulphur-Crested Cockatoo	*Cacatua sulphurea*	228 – 315
Greater Sulpur-Crested Cockatoo	*Cacatua galenta galenta*	500 – 1250
Moluccan cockatoo	*Cacatua moluccensis*	670 – 800
Roseate cockatoo	*Eolophus reseicapillus*	340 – 480
Umbrella cockatoo or Great white cockatoo	*Cacatua alba*	530 – 610
Blue and gold macaw	*Ara ararauna*	850 – 2000
Scarlet macaw	*Ara macao*	810 – 1100
Hahns macaw (Noble macaw)	*Ara nobilis*	150 – 180
Orange winged amazon	*Amazona amazonica*	440 – 470
Blue fronted amazon	*Amazona aestiva*	275 – 510
Yellow fronted amazon	*Amazona ochrocephala*	260 – 460
Double yellow headed amazon (Levaillant's)	*Amazona oratrix*	545
Mealey amazon	*Amazona farinosa*	600 – 685
Yellow billed amazon	*Amazona collaria*	215 – 270
Festive amazon	*Amazona festiva*	358 – 500
Hispaniolan amazon	*Amazona ventralis*	268
African grey parrot Three main varities with different average weights	*Psittacus erithacus*	310 – 460

Common name	Scientific name	Weight range in grams
Orange bellied Senegal parrot	*Poicephalus senegalus versten*	125 – 150
Dusky headed conure	*Aratinga acuticaudata*	155 – 185
Red masked parakeet	*Aratinga rubrolarvata*	158 – 168
Jendaya conure	*Aratinga jendaya (Eupisittula)*	118 – 128
Yellow rosella parakeet	*Platycercus flaveolus*	100 – 120
Pale headed rosella parakeet	*Platycercus adscitus palliceps*	100 – 120
Blue bonnet	*Psephotus heamatogaster*	100 – 120
Port lincoln	*Barnardius zonarius*	170 – 180
Blue headed parrot Pionus parrot	*Pionus menstrous*	238 – 278
Cockatiel	*Nymphicus hollandicus*	70 – 108
Budgerigar*	*Melopsittacus undulatus*	35 – 85
Bourke's parakeet	*Neophema bourkii*	50
Turquisine parakeet	*Neophema pulchella*	50
Blue winged grass parakeet	*Neophema chrysostoma*	38 – 50
Fischer's Lovebird	*Agapornis fischeri*	40 – 50
Order: **Columbiformes** Racing pigeon* ⎫ Feral pigeon* ⎭	*Columba livia*	230 – 540
Wood pigeon	*Columba palumbus*	454 – 680
Collared dove	*Streptopelia decaocto*	150 – 220
Diamond dove	*Geopelia cuneata*	40
Order: **Gruiformes** Moorhen	*Gallinula chloropus*	278
Coot	*Fulica atra*	520
Order: **Charadriiformes** Lapwing plover	*Vanellus vanellus*	200 – 235
Common sandpiper	*Tringa hypoleucos*	50

Common name	Scientific name	Weight range in grams
Herring gull*	*Larus argentatus*	750
Lesser black backed gull	*Larus fuscus*	675
Common gull*	*Larus Canus*	300 – 500
Black headed gull*	*Larus ribidundus*	175 – 295
Common/Arctic tern	*Sterna hirundo/parandisaea*	90 – 100
Heron*	*Ardea cinerea*	1362
Order: Proceilariiformes		
Fulmar petrel	*Fulmaris glacialis*	800
Order: Pelaecaniformes		
Gannet*	*Sula bassana*	2750
Shag	*Phalacrocorax aristotelis*	1700 – 2200
Order: Anseriformes		
Mute swan*	*Cygnus olor*	8000 – 13,000
Canada goose	*Branta canadensis*	4540
Domestic goose ⎫ Grey lag goose ⎭	*Anser anser*	3100 – 4090
Bean goose	*Anser arvensis*	2700 – 3600
Muscovy duck	*Cairina moschata*	3500 – 5000
Domestic duck ⎫ Mallard duck ⎭	*Anas platyrynchos platyrynchos*	975 – 3500
Shelduck	*Tadorna tadorna*	682
Order: Falconiformes		
Sparrow hawk*	*Accipiter nisus*	♂ 150 – 210 ♀ 190 – 300
Goshawk*	*Accipiter gentilis gentilis*	♂ 634 – 880 ♀ 980 – 1200
Buzzard*	*Buteo buteo*	680 – 1100
Red tailed hawk	*Buteo jamaicensis*	♂ 698 – 1147 ♀ 1000 – 1350
Harris' hawk	*Parabuteo unicinctus*	574 – 1000
Peregrine falcon	*Falco peregrinus*	♂ 560 – 850 ♀ 1100 – 1500

Common name	Scientific name	Weight range in grams
Kestrel*	*Falco tinnunculus*	♂ 145 – 167 ♀ 193 – 282
Saker falcon	*Falco cherrug*	♂ 680 – 990 ♀ 970 – 1300
Lanner falcon	*Falco biarmicus*	♂ 500 – 600 ♀ 700 – 900
Laggar falcon	*Falco jugger*	515
Merlin	*Falco columbarius*	♂ 160 – 170 ♀ 220 – 250

Order: Galliformes

Pheasant	*Phasianus colchicus*	♂ 1300 – 1600 ♀ 500 – 1135
Domestic chicken	*Gallus gallus*	1000 – 4000

Order: Strigiformes

Tawny owl*	*Strix aluco*	330 – 465
Short eared owl	*Asia flammeus*	325 – 440
Long eared owl	*Asia otus*	210 – 325
Little owl	*Athene noctua*	150 – 175
Eagle owl	*Bubo bubo*	1600 – 2500
Barn owl*	*Tyto alba*	262 – 600

Order: Passeriformes

Carrion crow*	*Corvus corone corone*	358 – 650
Rook	*Corvus frugilegus*	335 – 460
Jackdaw	*Corvus monedula spermologus*	145 – 210
Song thrush	*Tardus philomelos*	80
Blackbird*	*Turdus merula*	57
Robin*	*Erithacus rubecua*	20 – 30
Pekin robin	*Leothrix lutea*	26
Starling*	*Sturnus vularus*	64
Glossy starling	*Lamprotornis purpurus*	74 – 82
Great Indian hill mynah*	*Gracula religiosa intermedia*	180 – 260

Common name	Scientific name	Weight range in grams
House sparrow	*Passer domesticus*	25 – 30
Zebra finch*	*Poephila guttata*	10 – 16
Java sparrow*	*Padda oryzivora*	24 – 30
Gold finch	*Carduelis carduelis*	15 – 20
Cross bill*	*Loxia curvirostra*	41
Great tit*	*Parus major*	17.5 – 20.72
Blue tit*	*Parus caeruleus*	10 – 13.75
Green singing finch	*Serinus mozambicus*	10
Canary	*Serinus canaria*	12 – 29

2/Incubation and fledging periods of selected birds

Common name	Scientific name	Incubation period in days	Fledging period in days
Order: Psittaciformes			
Budgerigar	*Melopsittacus undulatus*	16 – 18	22 – 26
Australian parakeets in general	Genera *Neophema, Platycercus pseptotus Neopsephotus, Neomanodes*	18 – 19	30 – 45
Cockatiel	*Nymphicus hollandicus*	About 18	28
Ringneck parakeet	*Psittacula torquata*	23 – 24	55 – 65
Lorikeets	Genus *Trichoglossus*	25 – 26	62 – 70
Lovebirds	Genus *Agapornis*	About 18	30 – 35
Amazon parrots	Genus *Amazona*	23 – 24	45 – 60
Order: Columbiformes			
Domestic pigeon	*Columba livia*	17 – 19	35 – 37
Wood pigeon	*Columba palumbus*	17 – 19	16 – 38
Collared dove	*Streptopelia decaocto*	14	18 – 21
Order: Charadriiformes			
Herring gull	*Larus argentatus*	20 – 34	42
Common gull	*Larus canus*	24 – 27	35
Black headed gull	*Larus ribibundus*	22 – 24	35 – 42
Order: Anseriformes			
Mute swan	*Cygnus olor*	34 – 40	Leave nest in 24 – 48 hrs. Dependent on parents for 100 – 120 days
Grey lag goose ⎫ Domestic goose ⎭	*Anser anser*	24 – 30	Post fledging period: 53 – 57 days
Shelduck	*Tadorna tadorna*	28	45
Mallard	*Anas platyrynchos*	28	52
Pochard	*Aythya ferina*	23 – 29	49 – 56
Order: Falconiformes			
Sparrow Hawk	*Accipiter nisus*	32 – 35	24 – 30
Goshawk	*Accipiter gentilis gentilis*	36 – 38	41 – 43

Common name	Scientific name	Incubation period in days	Fledging period in days
Buzzard	*Buteo buteo*	34 – 38	42 – 49
Red tailed hawk	*Buteo jamaicensis*	32 – 35	43 – 48
Harris' hawk	*Parabute unicinctus*	33 – 36	40
Peregrine falcon	*Falco pergrinous*	35 – 42	35 – 42
Kestrel	*Falco tinnunculus*	28 – 31	27 – 30
Lanner falcon	*Falco biarmicus*	32 – 34	44 – 46
Golden eagle		41 – 49	about 77
Order: Galliformes			
Pheasant	*Phasianus colchicus*	21 – 28	Fly at 12 – 14 days
Domestic chicken	*Gallus gallus*	21	
Order: Strigiformes			
Tawny owl	*Strix aluco*	28 – 30	30 – 37
Short eared owl	*Asia flammeus*	24 – 28	24 – 27
Long eared owl	*Asia otus*	27 – 28	about 23
Little owl	*Athene noctua*	28 – 29	35 – 40
Barn owl	*Tyto Alba*	32 – 34	64 – 86
Snowy owl	*Nyctea scandiaca*	32 – 34	51 – 57
Order: Passeriformes			
Carrion crow	*Corvus corone corone*	16 – 20	26 – 38
Rook	*Corvus frugilegus*	16 – 18	29 – 30
Jackdaw	*Corvus monedula spermologus*	17 – 18	30 – 35
Magpie	*Pica pica*	17 – 18	22 – 27
Blackbird	*Turdus merula*	13 – 14	13 – 14
Song thrush	*Turdus philomelos*	13 – 14	13 – 14
Robin	*Erithacus rubecua*	13 – 14	12 – 14
Starling	*Sturnus vulgarus*	12 – 16	20 – 22
House sparrow	*Passer domesticus*	12 – 14	about 15
Zebra finch	*Poephila guttata*	12	14 – 21
Cross bill	*Loxia curvirostra*	12 – 13	17 – 25

Common name	Scientific name	Incubation period in days	Fledging period in days
Gold finch	*Carduelis carduelis*	12 – 13	13 – 14
Chaffinch	*Fringilla coelebs*	11 – 13	13 – 14
Great tit	*Parus major*	13 – 14	18 – 20
Blue tit	*Parus caeruleus*	17 – 18	about 16
Canary	*Serinus canaria*	13 – 14	Fed by parents for 28 days

3/Infectious diseases of birds: bacterial diseases

This table does not include all the diseases affecting poultry.

Disease	Cause	Species susceptible	Relative occurrence	Principal clinical signs*	Confirmation of diagnosis	Differential diagnosis*
Salmonellosis	Various species of *Salmonella* commonly *S. Typhimurium*. Carried by rodents, insects, water, wild birds.	All species. Wild birds often infected and carriers, particularly winter flocks.	Common except in raptors.	Sudden death or subacute septicaemic disease with enteritis. Chronic disease. PM signs depend on which stage died. Focal hepatic necrosis, caseous impaction of caeca localized necrosis of intestine. In pigeons often localizes in joints producing arthro-synovitis.	Isolation and culture of the organism. Serology. Fermentation of sugars.	A notifiable disease in the UK.
Avian Typhoid 'Pullorum Disease'	*Salmonella gallinarum*. *Salmonella pullorum*. Carrier birds.	Mainly diseases of poultry but can affect game birds and occasionally other birds including wild birds.	Common in insanitary conditions.	General malaise anorexia enteritis. In chronic form drop in egg production. At PM in *pullorum* infection disease localized in the ovary with misshapen ovules. PM of *gallinarum* cases shows septicaemic signs with enlarged liver and spleen.	Rapid slide agglutination. Test for *S. Pullorum*. otherwise as for other *Salmonella*.	

Disease	Cause	Species susceptible	Relative occurrence	Principal clinical signs*	Confirmation of diagnosis	Differential diagnosis*
Coli bacillosis	*Escherichia coli.*	All species.	Very common.	Often an acute septicaemic disease. In subacute or chronic form. PM shows air-sacculitis, fibrinous pericarditis with ecchymosis, a perihepatitis with enlarged liver. There may be hepatic granulomas. Enlarged necrotic spleen, caseous peritonitis. Organism often found in salpingitis and bumblefoot infections.	Isolation of the organism by culture.	*Mycobacterium avian* infection.
Tuberculosis	*Mycobacterium avium.*	All species. Wild birds, particularly starlings sparrows woodpigeons. Raptors. Anseriformes.	Not uncommon. Not uncommon. Common.	Debility, emaciation and diarrhoea. At PM tubercles can be found on and in any of the viscera, particularly the liver which may be studded with foci.	Stained smear from tubercles. Acid fast organisms shown by Ziehl – Neelsen's method. The tuberculin test is used in poultry for elimination of infected birds.	Pseudo-tuberculosis (*Yersiniosis*). Possibly confused with salmonellosis or *E. coli* at PM.

Disease	Cause	Species affected	Incidence	Clinical signs	Diagnosis	Differential diagnosis
			Not common nowadays.	Parrots have contracted disease from human contacts.		
Pseudo-tuberculosis	*Yersinia pseudo-tuberculosis* (Formerly called *Pasteurella pseudotuberculosis*). Organism carried by rodents and wild birds which contaminate food supplies.	All species. Wild birds, particularly those flocking in winter. Falciformes.	Not uncommon, particularly at the end of a severe winter. Rare.	No specific clinical signs in the live bird. At PM in the acute case the liver and spleen are enlarged. In the chronic condition there are yellowish white necrotic foci on the liver, spleen and pectoral muscles. There may be a severe enteritis.	Bacterial isolation by culture. No acid fast organism on Ziehl-Neelsen stained smear.	Tuberculosis. Sub acute fowl cholera.
Avian cholera	*Pasteurella Multocida* organism. Large numbers excreted in droppings and nasal discharge.	Most species. Wild Passeriformes. Owls. Diurnal raptors. Anseriformes. Galliformes.	Can cause epidemics in aviaries. Sporadic epidemics. Occasional. Uncommon. Common. Common.	A highly infectious and virulent disease often producing sudden death. Dyspnoea, mucoid oral discharge, diarrhoea. PM Septicaemic charges with multiple petechia.	Stained smear of liver imprints. Giemsa, Leishman's or methylene blue show bipolar stained rounded end rods. Culture and animal innoculation.	*E. coli.* Septicaemia. Pseudo-tuberculosis. Erysipelas.

Disease	Cause	Species susceptible	Relative occurrence	Principal clinical signs*	Confirmation of diagnosis	Differential diagnosis*
Anatipestifer infection	*Pasteurella anatipestifer* probably from the egg.	A specific infection of ducklings. Very occasionally other species of poultry.		Occular discharge, diarrhoea. Signs of central nervous disease. Often just found dead. PM congestion of lungs, enlarged liver and spleen. Fibrinous membranes on the viscera. Pericarditis and perihepatitis. Inspissated caseation in the air sacs.	Stained smear from lesions shows Gram-negative pleomorphic rods often in long filaments. Bacterial culture and isolation of the organism.	Duck plague. Viral enteritis. Duck viral hepatitis. Coccidiosis and as above for *P. multocida*.
Erysipelas	*Erysipelothrix insidiosa*.	All species. Pigeons.	Only occasionally seen but can cause epidemics in aviaries. Particularly susceptible.	Dullness, inappetence. Loose droppings. Septicaemic in a subacute form conjunctivitis may be seen in budgerigars.	Stained smear shows a Gram-positive pleomorphic slender rod like bacterium which is sometimes beaded.	As for avian cholera.
Listeriosis	*Listeria monocytogenes*.	Many species.	Rare.	Often a peracute septicaemia occasionally there is opisthotonus and other CNS signs. Sometimes produces a wasting disease.	Stained smear from liver and brain. Shows a Gram-positive coccobacillus. Culture.	

Anthrax.	*Bacillus anthracis.*	All species probably susceptible except vultures. Occurs if birds feed on infected meat or carrion.	Very rare. Usually in zoos.	Acute disease enlarged liver, spleen and kidneys. Areas of haemorrhage throughout the carcass.	Stained smear with methylene blue shows typical rod shaped baccilli.	Lead poisoning.
Botulism (Limberneck) 'Western Duck Sickness'	*Clostridium botulinum* 'C' toxin found in rotting carcasses and rotting vegetable and invertebrate matter.	Particularly Anseriformes also gulls and raptors feeding on carrion. Vultures are resistant to the toxin.	Not uncommon in hot, humid weather of late summer in UK.	A progressive flaccid paralysis of the neck, the legs and wings. Greenish diarrhoea due to anorexia. No PM signs.	Mouse protection inoculation test using specific antitoxin.	Poisoning with chlorinated hydrocarbons. Newcastle disease. In raptors hypocalcaemia. Listeriosis.
Avian Mycoplasmosis	*Mycoplasma* (P.P.L. organisms) Pleuropneumonia like organisms many strains may be commensals.	All species. Turkeys. Poultry and pheasants. Pigeons parrots Passeriformes. Diurnal raptors.	Very common. Common. Not uncommon. Occasional.	An upper respiratory infection, coryza, sneezing, sinusitis, blepharitis. In poultry affects the joints causing lameness. Clinical signs and PM are not pathognomonic. Often associated with other organisms such as *staphylococci, streptococci* and *E. coli.*	Culture of the causative organism. Serology only really applicable to poultry. Intracytoplasmic inclusions in impressions stained with Giemsa.	Often associated with other upper respiratory infections: Ornithosis Trichomoniasis.

* In many infectious diseases of birds the clinical signs are not pathognomonic and the disease can only be diagnosed on post-mortem and subsequent laboratory examination. When making a diagnosis please refer to the relevant organ system in the chapter on post-mortem technique.
Other bacterial organisms such as *staphylococci, streptococci, proteus, pseudomonas, corynebacterium* species act as secondary invaders but are not usually the prime cause of disease.

4/Infectious diseases of birds: viral/rickettsial infections

Disease	Cause	Species susceptible	Relative occurence	Principal clinical signs	Confirmation of diagnosis	Differential diagnosis
Ornithosis psittacosis chlamydiosis.	Various strains of chlamydia, rickettsial-like organisms.	All species particularly psittacines, Anseriformes. Columbiformes.	Not uncommon, Common.	Unthriftiness. Occular and nasal discharge, dyspnoea, enteritis. These signs are not pathognomic. PM hepatomegaly—patchy faint necrosis. Mottled enlarged spleen, air-sacculitis, pericarditis, sometimes serosal haemorrhage. One cause of 'one eyed cold' in pigeons.	Impression smears from liver. Stain modified Ziehl-Neelsen or Machiavello stain. Isolation by culture of the organism from faeces and tissues. Organism can be isolated from faeces of apparently healthy birds.	Pacheco parrot virus. Herpes virus of other species. Pox infection. Mycoplasmosis. Trichomoniasis often together with ornithosis. Salmonellosis. Avian influenza.
Pacheco's parrot disease.	Herpes virus. Asymptomatic carriers.	All Psittacines.	Not often diagnosed. May be more common than realized.	Often peracute may be just found dead with no premonitory signs. PM faintly mottled liver due to saucer-shaped necrotic areas. Sometimes necrotic focci in kidney and lungs.	Isolation of casual organism by culture in embryonated eggs.	Chlamydia infection.

Falcon inclusion body hepatitis.	Herpes virus	The virus is specific for diurnal raptors	A non-specific generalized disease. PM focal diffuse necrosis of the enlarged liver and spleen. May also show signs on the lungs and kidneys.	May be more common than generally realized	Avian tuberculosis. Newcastle disease.
Owl herpes virus	Herpes virus	Believed to occur only in the eared owls	May be peracute with sudden death. Necrotic foci in the oropharanx may look like Trichomoniasis which can also be a secondary invader. Necrotic foci in liver, spleen, intestine and lungs.		
Pigeon herpes virus.	Herpes virus	Specific for pigeons	Mainly respiratory, dyspnoea, rhinitis, conjunctivitis. Sometimes CNS signs with tremors and ataxia. PM may show faint necrotic foci in liver and other viscera. Diptheroid membrane in pharynx and larynx.	All these viruses are closely related serologically. The viruses can be isolated in embryonated eggs. Histopathology shows nuclear inclusion bodies from the areas of necrotic foci of liver and spleen	Paramyxo virus in pigeons
Crane herpes	Two distinct viruses	Cranes	Apathy and diarrhoea		As above
Ciconiae herpes		Storks	Both viruses cause lesions in the liver, spleen, kidney and intestine.		

Disease	Cause	Species susceptible	Relative occurrence	Principal clinical signs	Confirmation of diagnosis	Differential diagnosis
Amazon tracheitis.	Herpes virus.	Amazon parrots.	?	Pseudomembranous tracheitis. Chronic dyspnoea with rales.	Isolation of the causal organism in chicken embryo—chorio-allantois.	Avitaminosis A. Newcastle disease.
Infectious laryngotracheitis.	Herpes virus.	Chickens. Pheasants. Peafowl.	Not common because of vaccination.	*Acute form* respiratory signs with death in 2 to 3 days. PM haemorrhage tracheitis. *Sub acute form.* Respiratory signs less severe. *Chronic form* cough only if stressed. PM mucoid diphtheritic membranes on the upper respiratory tract with a cheesy like necrosis.	Inclusion bodies found in diseased tissue in the early stages. Growth of virus in chick embryo. Serum neutralization tests.	Chronic fowl pox. Avitaminosis A. Newcastle disease.
Duck plague. Duck viral enteritis.	Herpes virus. Resevoir in wild water fowl.	Ducks. Geese. Swans.	Sporadic outbreaks.	Peracute – often just found dead. Blood from natural orifices. PM Haemorrhagic eruptive lesions of the gastro intestinal mucosa. Diphtheritic oesophagitis which is diagnostic.	Growth of the virus in chick embryo.	Bacterial septicaemia. Avian cholera. Erysipelas Duck virus hepatitis.

Disease	Nature / Cause	Species affected	Incidence	Clinical signs & PM	Diagnosis	Differential diagnosis
Marek's disease.	Herpes virus living in cells of feather follicle. Remains in feather debris for a long time.	Occurs in domestic fowl in birds as young as 6 weeks. Pigeons, possibly canaries. Has been reported in some wild birds.	Prior to vaccination very common. Rare.	Progressive paresis and paralysis leading to emaciation. PM lymphoid infiltration of viscera, thickening of the peripheral nerves.	Clinical signs combined with post-mortem picture.	Avian leukosis. Riboflavin deficiency causes thickening of the nerves in young chicks.
Leucosis complex.	A number of RNA viruses of the leucosis/sarcoma group.	All species.	Rare.	Tumours particularly of the liver (Big Liver disease) but also of the kidney, spleen and skin.	PM macroscopic lesions.	Marek's disease.
Newcastle disease. (*A notifiable disease in the U.K.*)	Parmyxo virus serotype Group I.	All species. Galliformes (very susceptible). Anseriformes (not very susceptible). Raptors (not very susceptible). Passeriformes, psittacines—both have a variable susceptibility. Columbiformes. Fairly resistant to serotype Group I.	Not uncommon. Rare. Not very common. True Newcastle disease is rare.	Respiratory signs with rhinitis and conjunctivitis; gastrointestinal signs with greenish, watery diarrhoea. Central nervous signs—torticollis, opisthotonus, dropping of a wing, paralysis. PM sometimes petechia on viscera and green staining around the vent.	Virus isolation and haemaglutination – inhibition test.	1) Avian Pox. 2) Laryngo tracheitis. 3) Falcon, crane pigeon, owl, ciconiae herpes virus infections. A notifiable disease in the UK. B vitamin deficiencies. Listerosis. Paramyx virus. Disease of pigeons.

Disease	Cause	Species susceptible	Relative occurrence	Principal clinical signs	Confirmation of diagnosis	Differential diagnosis
Paramyxo disease.	A mutant strain of P.M.V. – 1.	Only identified in pigeons at present.	Common if not vaccinated.	Signs similar to Newcastle disease but mainly those of the central nervous system which start before any diarrhoea is seen, no signs of respiratory disease.	Haemaglutination inhibition test and virus isolation.	Pigeon herpes virus.
Avian Pox.	Avian Pox viruses. At least 17 distinct viruses identified, each adapted to different families of birds. These viruses often transmitted by arthropod vectors.	Most species susceptible to a specific virus.	Common in Passeriformes more common in S. American parrots than Australian parrots. Uncommon raptors.	Acute form: septiocemic sudden death, Usual in canaries. Sub acute to chronic form: yellowish papules changing to brown appear on the skin of head and legs. Conjunctivitis, erythema, oedema, lachrymation, dysphagia because diphtheric lesions appear in oropharanx, if diphtheric membranes removed—bleeding	Histopathology. Bollinger bodies—intracytoplasmic inclusions seen in the epithelium of the skin.	Avitaminosis A. Newcastle disease. Largotracheitis. Amazon tracheitis.

Disease	Cause	Species	Incidence	Signs	Diagnosis	Notes
Avian influenza. Fowl plague.	Influenza 'A' viruses. A number of serotypes.	Galliformes ducks and other Anseriformes. Psittacines Not seen in pigeons.	Uncommon. Not in UK since 1979. Rare.	An inapparent sinusitis to a severe respiratory disease.	Virus isolation and serology.	Ornithosis. Newcastle disease. Fowl cholera.
Duck virus hepatitis.	Picorna virus spread in faeces.	Ducklings from 2 weeks of age.	Not uncommon.	Peracute. Sudden death within hours. Maybe sluggishness then CNS signs e.g. opisthotonus PM Liver enlarged and shows petechial haemorrhages.	Innoculation of the embryonated chicken egg.	Often secondarily infected with *Salmonella*. Duck virus enteritis. Bacterial septicaemias. Coccidiosis. Mycotoxicosis.

Disease	Cause	Species susceptible	Relative occurrence	Principal clinical signs	Confirmation of diagnosis	Differential diagnosis
Goose virus hepatitis. Goose influenza. Goose plague.	Parvo virus.	Goslings.	Not uncommon.	Coryza, diarrhoea, ataxia. PM fibrinous exudate of viscera. Enlarged liver petechiae haemorrhages.		
Quail bronchitis.	An adeno virus. Poultry harbour virus.	Bob white quail.	Game bird farms in N. America.	Acute onset coughing, sneezing, tracheal rales Occasional CNS signs mortality 50–80%. PM excess mucus in airways, cloudy air sac membranes.		
Eastern and western equine encephalitis and other encephalitis.	Arboviruses transmitted by biting insects. Mainly in the Americas but also in other parts of the world.	Birds may act as important hosts. All species. Galliformes, Passeriformes, Anseriformes most susceptible.	Possibly common carriers in birds. Clinical disease in birds rare.	May cause CNS signs in birds, i.e. paralysis and incoordination.		
Specific avian encephalomyelitis. Epidemic tremor.	Picornavirus.	Mainly a poultry disease, can affect pigeons and Anseriformes.	Affects young chicks 1 – 2 weeks.	CNS signs—epidemic tremors paralysis, incordination. Fall in egg production in older birds.	Innoculation of embryonic eggs and serology.	Newcastle disease. Marek's disease.

Other less well understood viral-like conditions

Budgerigar herpes virus.		Budgerigar.		Reduced hatchability and may be associated with *'Feather Duster' syndrome.*	
Cockatoo beak and feather syndrome.	Probably a virus.	Probably all old world psittacines.	Not uncommon.	Loss of normal contour feathers replaced by abnormal plumage, i.e. short club-like feathers fret lines in the vane, constrictions on the shaft, curled feather. Feather retained in blood-filled sheath. Beak becomes more shiny, elongated, shows fault lines, surface flakes off.	Histopathology.
Papova virus.	A papova-like agent reported by Bernier (1981).	Nestling budgerigars 1 – 15 days of age Similar syndromes seen in other psittacines	May be more common than realized.	Abdominal distension lack of down feathers on back and abdomen. Hydropericardium. Enlarged heart. Enlarged liver. Ascites. Liver shows multiple white or yellow spots.	

229

5/Infectious diseases of birds: mycotic diseases.

Disease	Cause	Species susceptible	Relative occurence	Principal clinical signs	Confirmation of diagnosis	Differential diagnosis
Aspergillosis.	*Aspergillus fumigatus.*	All species captive and wild.	Common.	Can be peracute, usually chronic debility with various respiratory signs. PM yellowish miliary nodules in the lungs. Disclike plaques of grey, necrotic material in the respiratory tract and sometimes in the alimentary canal. Lesions may occur on the air sacs and may be granulomatous.	Examine necrotic foci for signs of hyphae and fruiting bodies. Use 20% potassium hydroxide and stain with lactophenol blue. Radiography, laparoscopy, tracheal swabs for culture and cytology.	Tuberculosis. Pseudo-tuberculosis. Pox virus. Trichomoniasis. *E. coli.*
Candidiasis (Moniliasis).	*Candida albicans* (Monilia). May occur in normal gut flora and overgrow after indescriminate use of antibiotic and bad hygiene.	Pigeons, turkeys, partridges, grouse, budgerigars, psittacines, Passeriformes.	Not uncommon. Said to be common in nectar-feeding birds.	Vomiting, loss of condition, sporadic deaths. PM mucosa of crop and oesophagus thickened and covered in a soft whitish cheesy material under which the mucosa is velvet-like.	It is possible to examine the crop in a live bird with a laparoscope. Wet mount smears stained with lactophenol blue, Gram stain, methylene blue or Giemsa show yeast like organisms.	Trichomoniasis. Sour crop causing a bacterial necrosis. *Salmonella typhimurium* in passerines can infect the crop. In psittacines physiological malfunction and hypertrophy.

					Mange mite infection.
Dermatomycosis (Ringworm) (Favus).	*Trichophyton* species. *Gladosporium* species.	Probably occurs in all species but particularly Passeriformes.	Uncommon.	Loss of feathers. Skin thickened; greyish-white, lifeless. Skin has tendency to be corrugated and encrusted.	Microscopical examination of skin scrapings. Histopathology. Culture.
Actinomyces.	Reported by Coffin in parrots. One case seen by the author in a Moluccan cockatoo which formed a granuloma caudal to the vent.	Uncommon.		Histopathology and culture.	

Crytococcus neoformans and mucor infections have been diagnosed [Woerpel & Rosskopf (1984)].

6/Parasitic diseases of birds: protozoal parasites.

Disease	Cause	Species susceptible	Relative occurence	Principal diagnostic signs	Confirmation of diagnosis	Differential diagnosis
Coccidiosis.	A large number of host-specific protozoal parasites which invade the mucosa of the intestine; most belong to the genus *Eimeria*.	Poultry and game birds.	Common.	Mild to severe diarrhoea sometimes blood stained. General unthriftiness anaemia.	Identification of the oocysts by routine faecal flotation methods.	
		Raptors.	Probably not pathogenic.	PM, the lesions occur in specific parts of the intestine in poultry according to the species of *eimeria*. Lesions are mostly congestion, haemorrhage and often excess mucus. Sometimes white spots are seen on the wall of the gut. In geese the kidneys may be enlarged with white necrotic areas.		
		Parrots.	Occasional.			
		Passerines.	Very rare.			
		Anseriformes. Some species invade the kidneys of anseriformes and owls.	Not uncommon.			
	Isospora species are not so host-specific and generally not pathogenic.		Common in many wild birds.			

232

Disease	Organism	Species affected	Incidence	Clinical signs / PM	Diagnosis	Remarks
Trichomoniasis. 'Frounce'. 'Canker'.	*Trichomonas gallinae.*	Probably all species. Possibly many healthy carriers occur. Raptors. Pigeons. Parrots.	May be more common than realized. Not uncommon. Common. Uncommon.	Inappetence, dyspnoea un-thriftiness. Often consider-able loss of weight. PM, yellowish-white cheesy material often quite thick found anywhere from the oropharanx to the proventri-culus. Initially the lesions may be quite small but latterly may become gross.	Microscopical examination of the lesions for the highly motile parasites. If in doubt culture in a special liquid medium overnight. Before examining, warm the slide.	*Candidiasis* Vitaminosis A.
Giardiasis.	*Giardia intestinalis.*	Reported in many species of birds and mammals including man.	Very rare in birds.	Chronic diarrhoea and unthriftiness.	Identification of the motile parasites which can be difficult. Cysts can be seen by using flotation methods.	May be associated with concurrent *E. coli.* Coccidiosis.
Hexamitiasis.	*Hexamita meleagridis.*	Young birds turkeys, pigeons, pheasants, quail, peafowl.	Not very common.	Diarrhoea and unthriftiness. PM, catarrhal inflammation of the intestine.	Histopathology Demonstration of active parasites in droppings.	Trichomoniasis and giardiasis.

Disease	Cause	Species susceptible	Relative occurrence	Principal clinical signs	Confirmation of diagnosis	Differential diagnosis
Histomoniasis 'Blackhead'.	*Histomonas meleagridis* organism carried by ova of the worm *Heterakis gallinae* which acts as a vector.	Turkeys and other gallinaceous birds. chickens, pheasants, quail, peafowl, grouse.	Common, particularly if the birds associate with the domestic fowl which carry the vector.	Dullness—diarrhoea with yellowish droppings. PM Caeca enlarged, filled with caseous necrotic material. Characteristic cream-coloured circular lesions on the liver the centre of which is darker and haemorrhagic.	PM lesions and histopathology.	
Lankesterellosis.	*Lankesterella* species invade the lymphocytes and monocytes of birds. Red mites may act as vectors.	Probably all species of Passeriformes.	Probably more common than realized.	Usually non-pathogenic. Very heavy infections may cause death in young birds, particularly nestlings.	Examination of stained smear from blood, liver spleen and bone marrow. Parasites *non-pigmented* within the lymphocytes. Difficult to find in peripheral blood.	*Plasmodium. Haemoproteus.*
Avian malaria.	*Plasmodium* species invade red blood cells of the bird. Transmitted by blood sucking arthropods.	Probably most species of birds The parasite is not always host specific.	May be more common than realized, although rarely pathogenic.	Swelling of the eyelids reported in some species Depression, fluffed up feathers, anaemia. Death within a few hours. Probably only important in canaries and penguins kept in warm climates.	Examination of stained smear of blood for the *pigmented* parasites within the erythrocytes.	Haemoproteus infection. Leucocytozoonosis infection.

Disease	Parasite / transmission	Hosts	Frequency	Pathogenicity	Diagnosis	Other names
Leucocyto-zoonosis.	*Leucocytozoon* species. Transmitted by biting flies (*Simulium*) and midges (*Culicodes*).	Domestic fowl. Anseriformes. Passeriformes. } Psittacines. Owls.	Common in right weather conditions. Rare. Common.	Anorexia, anaemia. Disease only occurs if conditions are right for build up of flies. Important disease of ducks and geese in N. America where the black fly (*Simulium*) is prevalent.	Examination of stained blood. Large parasites may be seen to have invaded usually the leucocytes but sometimes red blood cells.	Avian malaria. Haemoproteus infection.
Haemoproteus.	*Haemoproteus* species transmitted by hippoboscid flat flies, mosquitoes, midges.	Galliformes, Passeriformes, Columbiformes, many wild. Psittacines. Owls. Falciformes.	Common. Not very common. Common. Quite common.	Not usually pathogenic except in a heavy infection.	Examination of stained blood smear shows pigmented parasites *within* the red blood cells. May be confused with plasmodium infections.	Avian malaria. Leucocytozoonosis.
Trypanosomiasis.	*Trypanosome* species. Biting anthropods.	Passeriformes, Galliformes, Anseriformes, Columbiformes, Strigiiformes, Falciformes.	Probably not uncommon.	Probably not pathogenic.	Examination of a stained smear of blood or bone marrow. Parasite occurs in the plasma.	

Other protozoal parasites that occur in birds: *Toxoplasma*; *Sarcocystis* infection; *Aegyptianella Piroplasmosis* infection.

7/Parasitic diseases of birds: helminth parasites

Disease	Cause	Species susceptible	Relative occurence	Principal clinical signs	Confirmation of diagnosis	Differential diagnosis
Ascaridiasis.	Ascaridia (a) Galli (b) Hermaphrodita (c) Columbae	Psittacines. Domestic fowl and game birds. Passeriformes. Falciformes. Columbiformes.	Not uncommon. Quite common. Rare. Not uncommon. Common.	Loss of condition. Sudden death due to impaction of the bowel said to cause paralysis of the legs because of impaction of the intestine in parakeets.	Examination of the droppings by normal flotation methods show typical worm eggs.	
Gizzard and intestinal worms.	*Porrocaecum* species.	Passeriformes ducks.		**Unthriftiness. PM Larvae** found under horny lining of gizzard and worms may cause tumours in serosal surface of intestine.	PM signs.	
Proventricular and gizzard worms.	*Spiroptera* species (*Habronema*). Ground-living arthropods.	Galliformes. Passeriformes. Psittacines.	May be more common than realized.	Parasite burrows beneath the horny lining of the gizzard and into the mucosa of oesophagus and intestine. General unthriftiness and sudden death.	Examination of droppings for embryonated eggs.	

Gizzard worms of ducks and geese.	*Amidostomun anseris* Adult birds act as carriers.	Ducks and geese domestic and wild.		Anorexia, emaciation in goslings and ducklings— death. Erosion (and necrosis) of lining of gizzard, larvae found beneath the lining. May attack proventriculus and oesophagus.	PM signs.
Capillariasis (Threadworms) (Hairworms).	*Capillaria* species sometimes pass through the secondary host the earthworm.	Galliformes. Passeriformes. Strigiformes. Psittacines. Falciformes.	Not uncommon.	Loss of condition, lack of appetite, mucoid diarrhoea eventually death. PM in heavy infection anaemia. Worms found in lumen of intestine, oesophagus and buccal cavity, (in owls) worms burrow into mucosa.	Examination of droppings shows eggs of the parasite with typical bi-polar plugs. Eggs shed sporadically, therefore, examine serial specimens. Trichomoniasis in raptors. Examine scrapings of mucosa of oropharanx for eggs.
Caecal worms carriers of the parasite *Histomonas*.	*Heterakis gallinae*. Earthworms act as a vector.	Domestic fowl and all gallinaceous birds Anseriformes.	Common.	The worm by itself is probably not pathogenic unless there is heavy infestation when there is unthriftiness and diarrhoea. Pin-point haemorrhages and nodules in mucosa of caeca.	Examination of the faeces for the ova which are not unlike those of *Ascaridia galli*, but the egg wall is slightly thinner.

Disease	Cause	Species susceptible	Relative occurrence	Principal clinical signs	Confirmation of diagnosis	Differential diagnosis
Syngamiasis (Gapes).	*Syngamus* species. Direct transmission or may pass through a transport host such as earthworms, slugs, snails.	Probably can infect all species and naturally occurs in many species.	Not uncommon. Very easy to find in many wild Passeriformes.	Dyspnoea—gaping, cough, shaking head. Anorexia, loss of condition death. PM parasites found in the trachea which may be completely blocked. Tracheitis, bronchitis, pneumonia.	Examination of the droppings for the typical egg with operculum at each end like a *Capillaria* egg but larger. Endoscopy in large birds of the trachea. Sometimes worms can be seen by naked eye.	*Capillaria* in raptors. Trichomoniasis. Candidiasis. *Aspergillus*. Avian pox.
Filiariasis.	Larvae of *Serrato spiculum tendo*. Found as micro filariae in blood stream. Biting arthropods act as vectors.	Falcons. Other species found in Passeriformes, psittacines.	Common in the tropics. May be found in imported birds. Not uncommon.	The larvae in the blood stream are of doubtful pathogenicity. However during body migration the larvae can cause quite a severe reaction in the lung and air sacs. The adult worm is found in the body cavities beneath the intestine, beneath the serosa, it is long thin and coiled.	Examination of a stained blood smear or a wet mount unstained blood smear to see the living micro filiarae. Examine the droppings for the embryonated egg which is oval-shaped like that of sygamus.	In the blood Do not confuse with trypanosomiasis.
Thorny headed worms.	Various species of acanthocephalids. All have intermediate invertebrate hosts.	Waterfowl. Passeriformes. Raptors.	Not very common.	Found in the mucosa of the intestine causing enteritis and unthrifiness if they are present in large numbers.	It may be possible to find the spindle shaped embryonated egg in the droppings. The	

Tapeworms.	A very large number of species of *Cestoda*. All require a secondary host—usually an invertebrate but may be fish.	Probably all species. Less common in the seed- and fruit-eating birds except in nestlings.	Not uncommon.	Not often pathogenic. General debility and diarrhoea, anorexia. PM varying degrees of enteritis together with the worms. If much mucus is present scrape the mucosa and examine the scrapings microscopically.	embryo contains a circlet of hooks on the head. Difficult to identify for the non-specialist. Finding the proglottids in the faeces. Examine more than one sample of droppings. *Railietina* species can produce nodules in gut wall which can be seen from the serosal surface and look like TB.
Flukes.	Numerous trematode species. Always require a secondary host such as a mollusc which is usually but not always aquatic.	Passeriformes.	Not very common.	Clinical signs indefinite. General unthriftiness. Signs depend where the flukes are located in the body. At PM they can be found in almost any part of the body	Finding fluke eggs in the droppings. PM signs.
		Waterfowl and aquatic birds.	Not uncommon.		
		Columbiformes.	Not common.		
		Falconiformes.	Most common in tropical areas and tend to be regionally located.		

8/Parasitic diseases of birds: arthropod ectoparasites.

Disease	Cause	Species susceptible	Relative occurence	Principal clinical signs	Confirmation of diagnosis	Differential diagnosis
Lice.	Biting or chewing lice (Mallophaga).	Probably all species. Lice are host specific. More than one species of lice may be found on the same bird.	Very common particularly in birds debilitated from other causes.	Most lice feed on feather debris and not blood. Cause irritation and restlessness. Healthy birds keep lice in check when preening, but heavy louse infection may lead to feather plucking.	Finding the lice or the eggs in the feathers. Often seen in anaesthetized birds and in recently dead birds.	
Hippoboscids (flat or louse flies).	Arthropods related to the 'Sheep Ked'.	Probably all species. Seen particularly in raptors, pigeons, swifts, martins, swallows.	Common on many wild birds.	Suck blood and may transmit *Haemoproteus*. Often jump onto human handler and can get into clothing and hair and remain some time. Has been recognized as a problem for sometime in nestling pigeons.	Recognition of the dorso ventrally flattened stout flies which may or may not have wings depending on the species.	
Fleas.	Many species of *Siphonaptera*.	Probably all species .	Not often seen. Can build up in nesting areas and nest boxes.	Irritation, restlessness. Although they suck blood they are of doubtful pathogenicity. They are not	Identification of adult eggs and larvae in nesting sites.	

Red mites. Northern fowl mite.	*Dermanyssus gallinae* *Ornithonyssus sylviarum*	Domestic poultry. Passeriformes. Columbiformes. Psittacines. Raptors.	Common. Not uncommon.	host specific so that birds can become infected with mammalian species from domestic pets. Can live on humans. Cause intense irritation and restlessness. Suck blood and cause anaemia and debility. *D. gallinae* only found on the bird at night. Hide in crevices during the day.	Examine perches and woodwork by torch light at night. Keymer (1969) suggests covering cage with a white cloth at night when mites can be seen on or under surface in the morning.	Red mite and northern fowl mite infection.
Harvest mites.	Larvae of *Trombicula* and other species, during spring and autumn.	Most ground living species.	Widespread clinical infection uncommon, localized.	Irritation may show vesicles where a bird has been biting. The adult mites may be quite large and are free living in woods, scrubland and old pasture. They feed on invertebrates and plants.	Identification of larvae on the skin.	

Disease	Cause	Species susceptible	Relative occurrence	Principal clinical signs	Confirmation of diagnosis	Differential diagnosis
Forage mite	Many species	Anywhere where food is badly stored in humid conditions.	Very common. May occur in huge numbers.	Not pathogenic but may be confused with the pathogenic mites. Causes considerable spoiling of grain and seed foods. May cause allergic reaction and very occasionally death after eating infected food. The author has seen a massive infestation of grain fed to over 100 quail with no deaths in the birds.	Very small. Off-white in colour.	
Air sac mites.	*Sternostoma* species.	Mostly reported in Passeriformes but occasionally psittacines.	Possibly more common than realized.	Loss of condition, dyspnoea, loss of voice, sneezing, gasping, death. PM Mites black in colour seen in trachea and upper air passages and in the air sacs.	They have been seen in the air sacs by laparoscopy.	Syngamus. Aspergillosis. Avian pox.
Scaly face and scaly leg mites. 'Depluming itch' or 'Feather rot' in pigeons.	*Knemidocoptes* species.	Budgerigars. Crossbills. Other species of psittacines. Canaries. domestic poultry. Wild birds.	Common. Common on legs. Occasional.	Grey-white encrustations around the cere, the beak, the commissures of the upper and lower beak often gross distortion of the beak. Tassle foot lesions on canaries and other passeriformes.	Mites easily identified in powdery scrapings. Clear slide with 10% KOH.	Carcinoma of beak. Avian pox. Papillomas of the legs.

Non-pathogenic feather mites occur in many birds and are found in the plumage feeding on feathers and skin debris. Quill and feather follicle mites may cause irritation and loss of feathers. Can be expressed from the quills of growing feathers, i.e. those in 'the blood'. Other non-pathogenic cytoditid mites, white in colour, are sometimes seen in the respiratory passages, air sacs and other organs of the body.

Ticks.	Ixodes ricinus and a number of other species.	Probably all species.	Uncommon. Most likely to be seen in birds recently imported from the tropics.	Irritation, loss of condition, anaemia and death if the infestation is severe. Small birds do not need many ticks to lose quite a lot of blood.	Identification of the parasite.
Dipterous flies.	Calliphora lucilia phormia species. All cause blow fly strike.	All species.	Not common but can invade gangrenous wounds or chicks in a dirty nest.	Typical signs of maggots.	

Mosquitoes, gnats, midges and black flies all bite and suck avian blood and often transmit blood parasites.

9/Poisons likely to affect birds

General comment. This list is not comprehensive and is only a guide. A specific diagnosis of poisoning is not often possible—much depends on circumstantial evidence. The analysis of samples can be expensive and the analyst must be given a good idea of what to look for. Many poisons do not cause acute death but in sublethal doses may be responsible for lower fertility, reduced resistance to infection and non-specific symptoms such as sporadic nervous tremors. Few cases of poisoning are malicious; most are due to carelessness or thoughtlessness.

Type of poison	Comments
Agricultural and gardening chemicals. Seed dressings and storage preservatives. Orgamomercury compounds.	Many substances are used to control infection of the seed and growing plant by micro-organisms. They may also be used to control weevils in stored grain. The chemicals may be used at the wrong dose or the treated seed inadvertently fed to birds. Supplies of many seeds come from countries where the control of these chemicals is not strict enough.
Insecticidal and herbicidal sprays. Agricultural fertilizers. Ammonium sulphate; phenoxyacid herbidices; carbamates and phosphorothionates.	Most notorious of the insecticides in the past are DDT and the polychlorinated biphenyls. Nowadays many organophosphates are used to spray growing crops including fruit farms. The cloud of spray may be blown by wind. The insects killed and contaminated with the insecticide may be eaten by birds. Nitrogenous fertilizers may leach into water supplies. Roadside and garden herbage may be contaminated by many chemicals. Water supplies of birds may become contaminated.
Insecticides used to control infection in domestic animals.	Sheep dips and preparations to control fly strike in sheep may be misused. Many organophospates used on domestic pets as sprays and baths are toxic if misused on birds.
Rodenticides.	In the past strychnine, arsenic, thallium, zinc phosphide and phosphorus were widely used and are still used in some countries. Warfarin and related compounds together with the organophosphates are now commonly used and birds may gain access to treated bait. Sodium fluoroacetate and fluoroacetamide are also widely used in many parts of the world and are very poisonous.

Molluscicides.

These are used to control garden pests and the vectors of many helminth infections. Metaldehyde and copper sulphate are both toxic to birds.

Alphachloralose.

These are used to control pigeons in urban areas. Affected pigeons are narcotized and may be eaten by raptors. Also used as a rodenticide.

Wood preservatives.

Bitumen paint, pentachlorophenol, creosote and naptha compounds may be used to preserve the woodwork of aviaries. This may be chewed by psittacines which may acquire sublethal doses.

Disinfectants.

Phenols and cresols are often used far more concentrated than the manufacturers' recommendations. Can lie in pools in the bottom of aviaries and dry on perches, etc. The quaternary ammonium antiseptics are relatively non-toxic.

Lead.

Cage or aviary birds may be exposed to old lead paint. Waterfowl and game birds may pick up lead from ground which has been heavily shot over. Waterfowl may gradually accumulate lead from discarded fishermans' lead weights lying in the bottom mud of watercourses. Lead poisoning has also been seen in waterfowl near a rubbish tip containing lead car batteries. Old lead mining areas, lead smelting and industrial areas may be heavily contaminated. Plants and insects become contaminated.

Raptors may pick up subclinical lead levels from the tissues of prey species and also intact lead shot from their gizzards, Reiser & Temple (1980). The latter may or may not be voided in the casting of the raptor.

Carbon monoxide.

These fumes can come from a car left running in a garage or from a gas central heating boiler or gas water heater which is not functioning properly due to inadequate draught.

Fumes from a teflon non-stick cooking utensil.

If this dries and overheats toxic fumes can be produced. Other plastics if burnt can produce toxic fumes.

Type of poison	Comments
Naturally occurring toxins.	*Botulism:* mentioned under infectious diseases. Blow flies often attack meat infected with *Clostridium botulinum*, the maggots pick up the toxin and they may then be eaten by birds. Another cause are dead aquatic invertebrates in rotting vegetation. Sometimes associated with poisoning by blue green algae.
	Hemlock: seeds eaten by pigeons have caused fatalities.
	Yew leaves: may be eaten by game birds and poison them. All parts of the plants are very poisonous.
	Alfatoxin: first discovered in groundnuts affecting turkeys. The toxin is a metabolite of an *Aspergillus* fungus which can grow in badly stored grain or seed.
	Ergot (*Claviceps purpurea*) Infected grain. If eaten in large amounts they cause necrosis of the extremities.
Tannins and alkaloids contained in plants.	The leaves and twigs of rhododendron, azalea, laburnum and many other plants are toxic to herbivorous mammals and the bark may be toxic for birds. The leaves and bark of many trees contain low grade toxins such as tannins. These are bitter tasting and are part of the plants' natural defence systems against insects and vertebrates feeding on them. Perrins (1979) has shown that blue tit nestlings fed on mealworms containing tannins grow more slowly than nestlings fed on mealworms which do not contain tannins. This phenomenon could occur with many other plant substances taken in directly or indirectly by birds.

For a full discussion of the subject of poisoning in birds the reader is referred to three publications: *Bird Diseases* by Arnall and Keymer; *Veterinary Aspects of Captive Birds of Prey* by Cooper; *First Aid and Care of Wild Birds* edited by Cooper and Eley. See further reading list.

10/Schedule of wild bird releases by Jane Ratcliffe (1971 – 1984)*

Common name	Scientific name	Number received for treatment	Died or put to sleep	Unfit for release; retained for breeding	Number released	Number of short stay patients kept less than 3 months	†Number of long stay patients kept over 3 months	Number recovered after release and interval in months	Number sited and identified and interim in months
Kestrel‡	*Falco tinnunculus*	90	11	4	75	62	13	6 (0.3–9)	1 (seen for many years in release area)
Merlin§	*Falco columbarius*	2	—	—	2	1	1	—	—
Peregrine¶	*Falco peregrinus*	3	—	3	—	—	—	—	—
Sparrow-hawk**	*Accipter nisus*	8	2	—	6	3	3	1 (7)	3 {36 24 16
Buzzard††	*Buteo buteo*	7	1	1	5	4	1	2 (5) (4.5)	—
Barn owl‡‡	*Tyto alba*	26	2	1	23	13	10	8 (1–22)	—

Common name	Scientific name	Number received for treatment	Died or put to sleep	Unfit for release retained for breeding	Number released	Number of short stay patients kept less than 3 months	†Number of long stay patients kept over 3 months	Number recovered after release and interval in months	Number sited and identified and interim in months
Tawny owl[§§]	Strix aluco	40	6	1	33	27	6	4(1-14) (+1)	—
Short eared owl	Asio flammeous	7	3	—	4	2	2	—	—
Little owl[¶¶]	Athene noctua	13	2	2	9	4	5	—	—
Swift***	Apus apus	3	—	—	3	3	—	—	1 (seen for several weeks)
House martin***	Delicron urbica	2	1	—	1	1	—	—	—
Kingfisher	Alcedo atthis	1	1	—	—	—	—	—	—
Greater spotted woodpecker	Dendrocopos major	1	—	—	1	—	—	—	Visited bird table a number of times
Wood pigeon	Columba dalumbus	2	—	—	2	1	1	—	1 seen in area 3 weeks later

								Bred in nest box 4 months after release
Collared dove	*Streptopelia decaocto*	1	—	—	1			
Great crested grebe	*Podiceps cristatus*	1	1					
Red shank	*Triga totanus*	2	2					
Lapwing	*Vanelus vanelus*	1		1				
Oyster-catcher	*Haematopus ostralugus*	1		1				
Dunnock	*Prunella modularis*	1			1	1		
Treecreeper	*Certhia familiaris*	1		1	1	1		
Totals		213	32	12	169	123	42	21	9

* Jane Ratcliffe is a naturalist resident in Cumbria. Many of these birds were initially examined and treated by the author and the table is given here as an indication of the level of success that can be achieved with adequate veterinary treatment combined with a high standard of nursing. All the birds were B.T.O. ringed before release so they could be subsequently identified.

† Some of the long stay cases had damaged plumage and had to be retained until completely moulted.

‡ Some of these birds were recovered between 25 – 30 kilometres away after an interval of 6 – 9 months. Approximately 42 of these kestrels had been held illegally captive and 8 were received with jesses on their legs. Ten were young birds which had fallen from the nest.

§ A merlin's nest was found in the release area 2 months after release and assumed to be that of the released bird because of the scarcity of the species in that area.

' All these birds were received weeks or months after injury when healing had started to take place. There was either gross malformation of the bone or severe soft tissue damage often together with infection.

** The one sparrow-hawk recovered was found drowned 7 months after release. Of the three birds seen after release, they were seen for periods of between 16 months and 3 years in their particular territories after release.

†† Of the two birds recovered one was found shot 5 months alfter release, the other was hit by a train 8 weeks after release and 26 kilometres away. This bird, a female, had been seen displaying with a male bird.

‡‡ Of the eight barn owls recovered 2 were found drowned in cattle troughs and 3 were involved in road accidents. The longest time after release was 22 months; most recoveries were within 3–5 months. One bird was recovered 40 kilometres away. Fifteen of these birds were habituated to a barn before release and 3 pairs raised young.

§§ One of these tawny owls was recovered 8 years after initial release. It was known to have bred a number of times in a local nest box. After treatment a second time it was released.

'' Two of these little owls bred in an aviary before release when young and parents were released together.

***It is essential these insect feeders are hospitalized for the minimum time.

Of the total number of birds treated 44 had fractures and 21 of these were eventually released. 61 were received in poor or emmaciated condition and only needed good nursing before release. The total number of illegally captive raptors received for retraining and release was 68.

11/Glossary of terms used in the text together with the more common expressions used by falconers and other aviculturalists.

Alcidae A family of short-winged marine diving birds, the auks, included in the large order Charadriiformes.

altricial nestlings Newly hatched birds born blind, helpless and without true feathers although they are covered in down. These chicks are nidicolous or nest attached and are entirely parent dependent.

Anseriformes The order of birds containing the two families Anhimidae (screamers) and Anatidae (ducks, geese, swans).

Areidae The family of birds containing the herons, egrets and biterns.

ayre See **eyrie**.

bate, bating A falconer's term; fluttering or flying off the fist or an object.

bewits Short strips of leather by which bells are fastened to the legs.

block A cylindrical piece of wood to which the hawk is attached by a leash and upon which it can perch.

calling off Luring a hawk from an assistant at a distance.

casting Fur, feathers and bone being the indigestible part of a raptor's diet which are periodically ejected in the form of a pellet.

Charadriiformes The order of birds containing sixteen families of aquatic birds, prominent amongst which are Haematopodidae (oyster catchers), Charadriidae (plovers and lapwings), Scolopacidae (sandpipers) and Laridae (gulls and terns).

cockatiel The smallest member of the sub-family Cacatuinae (cockatoos) group of parrots and a popular pet bird.

Ciconiidae A family of long-legged birds, the storks.

Columdidae A large family of birds including the pigeons and doves.

Columbiformes The order of birds containing the Columbidae, the sandgrouse and the extinct dodos.

conspecific Of the same species.

coping A falconers' term meaning to cut off the sharp points of beak and talons.

covert feathers The smaller feathers which cover the base of the shaft of the main flight feathers.

Corvidae The family of birds included in the order of Passeriformes and which contains the crows, magpies and jays.

creance A falconers' term referring to long line attached to the swivel and used when 'calling off' (q.v.).

eyess or eyas A nestling hawk taken from the 'eyrie' or nest.

eyrie (Ayre) Nest of a bird of prey perched high up.

feake When a hawk wipes its beak on a perch after feeding.

fledging The growing period of a young bird until it is able to fly.

frounce Trichomoniasis of the oropharanx of a raptor.

Galliformes An order of birds containing seven families included in which are the Tetraonidae (grouse and ptarmigan), Phasinidae (pheasants, peacocks, partridges, quails and domestic fowl), and the Meleagridae (turkeys).

gallinaceous Pertaining to the order Galliformes.

graminivorous Grass and cereal eating.

granivorous Feeding on grain and seeds.

hack, flying at Young falcons recently taken from the nest are allowed to fly freely only coming back to the falconer to be fed.

hack back To train a captive hawk to hunt and sustain itself in the wild.

Haemotopodidae A family of seashore wading birds, the oyster catchers.

haggard A hawk which has been caught in the wild, after it has undergone its first moult and has got its adult plumage.

hard bills Birds that feed by cracking open seeds.

hood A leather hat placed over the head of a hawk to blindfold it and to make it more easy to handle.

hornbill Medium to large tropical bird with brightly coloured and large bill that is often surmounted by a large casque.

imping A falconer's method of repairing a broken flight or tail feather.

interremigial ligament An elastic ligament lying within the skin fold caudal to radius and ulna, carpus, metacarpus and digits of the wing. It unites the shafts of the primary and secondary feathers.

jack The male merlin (*Falco columbarius*).

jesses The short, narrow straps of leather fastened round a hawk's legs to hold it.

Laridae The family of birds containing the gulls and terns.

leash A long, narrow strip of leather attached via the swivel to the jesses (q.v.).

long-winged hawks The true falcons. The Falconidae including peregrine, saker, lanner, laggar, merlin and kestrel. See Appendix 1.

lure A flaconer's apparatus for recalling a hawk. A bunch of feathers wrapped around a piece of meat and weighted. Sometimes two wings tied together. It is swung by a cord in a large arc around the falconer.

lutino A yellow bird (usually psittacine) with no other markings and red eyes.

macaw A group of South American parrots. These are mostly, but not all, fairly large birds with a patch of bare skin on each side of the face.

manning Taming a hawk.

Megapodiidae The family of robust ground dwelling birds resembling pheasants found in S.E. Asia and Australia. Also known as incubator birds.

Mergus A genus of sea ducks.

mews A place where hawks are kept to moult (Mew v. to moult).

mules Hybrid canaries produced by crossing the canary with other finches such as goldfinches and greenfinches.

musket The male sparrow-hawk.

mutes The faeces of a hawk (mute v. to void faeces). Short-winged hawks (e.g. sparrow-hawk, goshawk.) are said to 'slice', i.e. eject the mutes horizontally.

ostringer (austringer) A falconer who flies short-winged hawks (e.g. goshawk).

pannel A falconer's term meaning the stomach of a hawk.

parakeet A small parrot. In the USA usually refers to the budgerigar.

Passeriformes The order of birds containing the largest number of species grouped into 55 families. It contains all the birds that have three forward toes and one well developed hind toe—an adaptation to perching.

passerines Pertaining to the order Passeriformes.

Phalocrocoracidae The family of birds containing the cormorants and shags.

Picidae The family of birds containing the woodpeckers.

pin feathers First sign of a developing feather, still retained within its sheath.

precocial chicks Newly hatched birds born covered in downy feathers, active and able to find their own food. These chicks are nidifugous or nest leaving.

prepatagial (propatagial) Referring to the prepatagium, a membranous fold of skin between the shoulder and carpal joints forming the leading edge of the wing.

primary feathers The main flight feathers attached to the metacarpal bones and digits.

Psittaciformes The order of birds containing one family—the psittacidae or parrots.

psittacines Parrots and related species.

Psittacula **parakeets** A large genus of medium-sized, mostly asiatic parakeets, including the popular plumheaded and ringnecked species.

Rallidae The family of birds known as rails including the coots, gallinules and moorhens.

Ramphastidae The toucans. S. American tropical birds with large brightly coloured bills.

raptor A bird with a hooked beak and sharp talons—a bird of prey.

redrump parakeet A species of small Australian parrot with red feathers over the base of the tail or rump.

remiges The main flight feathers of the wings (i.e. the primaries and secondaries).

short winged hawks Usually taken to mean the accipiters or bird hawks which inlude the goshawks and coopers hawk. Also refers to the broad winged birds—the buzzards.

soft bills Birds that feed on fruit or insects.

Spheniscisformes The order of birds containing the penguins.

split A heterozygous bird carrying a recessive colour.

stoop The swift descent of a falcon on the quarry from a height.

Sulidae The family of birds containing the gannets and boobies.

swivel Used to prevent the jesses and leash (q.v.) from becoming twisted when the hawk is tethered to its perch.

tiercel (tercel) The male of any species of hawk. The female is known as the falcon, especially the peregrine.

tiring A tough piece of meat or tendon given to a hawk to help exercise the muscles of the back and neck.

Turdidae The family of birds containing the thrushes and including such birds as the blackbird, the European robin and the nightingale.

Ulno carporemigial aponeurosis A triangular aponeurotic sheet of elastic tissue, lying on the ventral side of the wing, just caudal to the metacarpus and joining the bases of the shafts of the meta carpal primary feathers.

to wait on When a hawk soars above the falconer waiting for the game to be flushed.

to weather To place a hawk on a perch out in the open. Usually an area shielded from extreme weather is chosen.

weaver birds Small to medium sized passerine birds. Many species are gregarious and include the common house sparrow. Some species are popular aviary birds.

whydahs (Widow bird) A group of parasitic passerine (like cuckoos) allied to the weaver birds. The males usually have long tail feathers.

12/Alphabetical list of manufacturers and suppliers of drugs together with their products mentioned in the text.

Abbott Laboratories Ltd., Queensborough, Kent Mell 5EL
Tel: (0795) 663371
'Erythrocin suspension' (Erythromycin)
Animal Care Products, 3M Medical Products, St. Paul, Minnesota, U.S.A.
'Vetcast casting tape'
Aktiebolaget, Hisingeplast, Box 2143, 403 11 Gothenburg, Sweden.
'Plastic Padding'
Armour Pharmaceutical Company Ltd., Eastbourne, Sussex.
Tel: (0323) 2142
'Supramid' (Pseudo monofilament polyamide)
Arnolds Veterinary Products Ltd., 14 Tessa Road, Richfield Avenue, Reading, Berkshire RG1 8NF.
Tel: (0734) 54064/5
'Gentovet' (Gentamicin sulphate B.P.)
Bayer UK Ltd., Agrochem Division, Eastern Way, Bury St. Edmunds, Suffolk IP 32 7AH
Tel: (0284) 63200
'Negasunt' (Larvicidal & bacteriostatic wound powder)
'Rompun' (Xylazine)
'Yomesan' (Niclosamide B. Vet. C.)
Beecham Animal Health, Veterinary Department, Beecham House, Brentford, Middlesex TW8 9BD
Tel: 01-560 5151
'Clamoxyl' preparations (Amoxycillin)
'Penbritin' preparations (Ampicillin)
'Pyopen' (Carbenicillin sodium) medical preparation
'Ticar' (Ticarcillin disodium) medical infusion.
Behring Inst., Animal Health Division, Hoechst House, Salisbury Road, Hounslow, Middlesex TW4 6JH
'Haemacel'
Berk Pharmaceuticals Ltd., St. Leonards House, St. Leonards Road, Eastbourne, East Sussex BN21 3UU
Tel: (0323) 641144
'Marinol Blue'
'Pevidine'
'Retarbolin' (Nandrolin cyclohexylproprionate)
Bimeda UK Ltd., Gores Road, Kirkby Industrial Estate, Liverpool L33 7XS
Tel: (0515) 473711
'Atropine sulphate'.
Boehringer Ingelheim Ltd., Southern Industrial Estate, Bracknell, Berkshire RG12 4YS
Tel: (0344) 24600
'Bisolvon' (Bromhexine hydrochloride)
Boots Company PLC, Thane Road, Nottingham NG2 3AA
Tel: (0602) 56255
'Vita food'

Bristol Myers Pharmaceuticals, Station Road, Langley, Slough, Berkshire 3LS 6EB
Tel: (0753) 44266
'Kantrex' (Kanamycin sulphate) medical preparation.
Calmic, (Branch of Wellcome)
'Zyloric' (Allopurinol) medical preparation.
Carnation Ltd., Danesfield House, Medmenham, Marlow, Bucks SL7 2ES
Tel: (06284) 6021
'Build-up' (Convalescent food) medical pack.
Ceva Ltd., P.O. Box 209, 3 Rhodes Way, Watford, Hertfordshire WD2 4QE
Tel: (0923) 35022
'Erythrocin' preparations (Erythromycin)
'Spectam' preparations (Spectinomycin)
Chevita GmbH (W. Germany), Marketed by Univet 2 Ltd. 110 Churchill Road, Bicester, Oxon OX6 7XB
Tel: (08692) 41287
'Ascapilla' (Cambendazole)
'Gabbrocol' (Dimetridazole, paramomycine)
'Mycosan-T' (Erthromycine, arsanilic acid, amino acids, vits. trace elements)
'Tylosin+' (Tylosine, chlortetracycline, arsanilic acid, amino acids, vits. trace elements)
'Vitin' (Vitamins, trace elements, amino acids, sugars and fatty acids)
Ciba-Geigy Agrochemicals, Whittlesford, Cambridge CB2 4QT
Tel: (0223) 833621
'Araldyte'
'Ertilen' injection (Chloramphenicol)
'Respirot' (Respiratory stimulant)
'Sermix' (Reserpine)
Ciba Laboratories, Horsham, West Sussex RH12 4AB
Tel: (0403) 50101 (Medical Products)
'Rimactane' (Rifampicin) medical preparation.
Crown Chemical Co. Ltd., Stair House, Lamberhurst, Kent TN3 8DJ
Tel: (0892) 890491/5
'Coryzium' (Furazolidone)
'Lamb Tonic' (18 amino acids, B vitamins, glucose)
'Mebenvet' (Medendazole)
'Hypnodil'
'Spartakon'
C Vet Ltd., Minister House, Western Way, Bury St. Edmunds, Suffolk ID33 3SV
Tel: (0284) 61131
'Collovet' (Multiconstituent tonic)
'Multivet' injection (Vitamins A, D₃, E, B vitamins sorbic acid preservatives)
Cyanamide of Great Britain Ltd., Animal Health Division, Fareham Road, Gosport, Hampshire P013 0AS
Tel: (0329) 236131
'Aureomycin' preparations (Chlortetracycline)
Dales Pharmaceuticals Ltd., Snaygill Industrial Estate, Keighley Road, Skipton, North Yorkshire BD23 2RW
Tel: (0756) 61311
'GA.C. Ear Drops'

Duphar Veterinary Ltd., Solvay House, Flanders Road, Hedge End, Southampton SO3 4QH
Tel: (04892) 81711
'Duphalyte' (Multi amino acid, vitamin, electrolyte and dextrose solution)
'Nifulidone' (Furazolidone)
Elanco Products Ltd., Kingsclere Road, Basingstoke, Hampshire RG21 2XA
Tel: (0256) 53131
'Tylan 50 Injectable' (Tylosin in propylene glycol)
'Tylasol soluble' (Tylosin tartrate)
'Brietal sodium' (Methohexitone sodium)
Ethicon Ltd., P.O. Box 408, Bank Head Avenue, Edinburgh, Scotland.
'Vicryl'
Farley Health Products Ltd., Torr Lane, Plymouth, Devon PL3 5VA.
Tel: (0752) 701621
'Complan') Convalescent and invalid foods.
'Farlene')
Fisons Pharmaceuticals Ltd., 12 Derby Road, Loughborough, Leics. LE11 0BB
Tel: (0509) 263113
'Hyalase' (Hyaluronidase)
Glaxo Laboratories Ltd., (Medical Products) 891–995 Greenford Road, Greenford, Middlesex UB6 0HE
Tel: 01 422 3434
'Eltroxine' (Thyroxine sodium) Medical preparation.
Glaxovet Ltd., Breakspear Road South, Harefield, Uxbridge, Middlesex UB9 6LS
Tel: Ruislip 30266
'Ceporex' (Cephalexin)
'Crystapen' (Sodium benzylpenicillin B.P.)
'Dimycin'
'Grisovin' (Griseof Ivin)
'Saffan' (Alphaxalone-alphadolone)
'Streptovex'
'Oxytetrin injection' (Oxytetracycline)
Hexcel Medical Products, Catherine House, 63 Guildford Road, Lightwater, Surrey.
'Hexcelite'
Hoechst UK Ltd., Animal Health Division, Walton Manor, Walton, Milton Keynes, Buckinghamshire MK7 7AJ.
Tel: (090868) 2050
'Panacure 2.5% Suspension' (Fenbendazole)
'Alugan' preparations (Bromocyclen)
Imp Electronics, Caraway Road, Fulbourn, Cambridge CB1 5DU
'Imp' Respiratory Monitor supplied by Veterinary Instrumentation, 50 Broomgrove Road, Sheffield S10 2NA
Imperial Chemical Industries PLC Pharmaceuticals Division, Alderley Park, Macclesfield, Cheshire SK10 4TF
Tel: (0625) 582828
'Cetavlon' (Cetrimide B.P.)
'Fluothane' (Halothane)
'Fulcin'

'Hibitane' concentrate 5% (25% v/v chlorhexidine gluconate B.P.)
'Nemicide' (7.5% w/v levamisole hydrochloride B.P.)
'Sulphamezathine' solution 1:3 (Sulphadimidine B.P.)
Intervet Laboratories Ltd., Science Park, Milton Road, Cambridge CB4 4BH
  Tel: 0223 311221
  'Androject' (testosterone phenylpropionate)
  'Dexadreson'
  'Durateston' (4 testerone esters)
  'Oxytocin S' (Synthetic oxytocin)
  'S.A. 37' (Vitamins, amino acids, minerals and essential fatty acids)
  'Stat' (Gastro intestinal sedative without antibiotic)
Janssen Pharmaceutical Ltd., Chapel Street, Marlow, Bucks SL7 1ET
  Tel: (06284) 71744
  'Daktarin injection' (Miconazole-antifungal)
  'Mebenvet' (Mebendazole) marketed by Crown Chemicals.
  'Nizoral' (Ketoconazole) Medical preparation
  'Hypnodil' (Metomidate)
Kulzer and Co. GmbH, Bereich Technik, Frölingstrasse 29, Postfach 1749 D6380 Bad Homburg.
  Tel: (06172) 7021
  'Technovit' 6091
Labs Applied Biology Ltd., 91 Amhurst Park, London N16 5DR
  Tel: 01-800 2252
  'Ornimed preparations' (Seed impregnated with antibiotics and vitamins)
Leo Laboratories Ltd., Longwick Road, Princes Risborough, Aylesbury, Bucks HP17 9RP
  Tel: 944 (08444) 7333
  'Perlutex injection' (Medroxyprogesterone)
Eli Lilly & Co. Ltd., Kingsclere Road, Basingstoke, Hampshire RG21 2XA
  Tel: (0256) 3241
  'Keflex' (Cephalexin monohydrate) ⎤
  'Keflin' (Cephalothin sodium)   ⎬
  'Nebcin' (Tobramycin sulphate)   ⎦
May & Baker Ltd., Dagenham, Essex RM10 7XS
  Tel: 01 592 3060
  'Nuvamide' suspension (Sulphonamides, neomycin kaolin)
  'Emtryl' soluble (Dimetridazole B.P.)
  'Flagyl' (Metronidazole B.P.)
  'Flagyl S' (Metronidazole suspension) Medical preparation
Merrell Pharmaceuticals Ltd., Meadowbank, Bath Road, Hounslow, Middlesex TW5 9QY
  Tel: 01-759 2600
  'Rifadin' (Rifampicin)
MSD Agvet, Division of Merk Sharp & Dohme Ltd., Hertford Road, Hoddesdon, Hertfordshire EN11 9BU
  Tel: (0992) 467272
  'Thibenzole' suspension (Thiabendazole B.P. Vet)
  'Ivomec' (Ivermectin)
Mycofarm Ltd., London Road, Braintree, Essex CM7 8QH

Tel: (0376) 21721
'Amfipen' (Ampicillin B.P.)
'Engemvcin' 5% (Oxytetracycline hydrochloride B.P.)
Nicholas Laboratories Ltd., P.O. Box 17, 225 Bath Road, Slough, Berkshire
SL14AV
Tel: (0753) 23971
'Genticin' (Gentamicin sulphate)
Norwich-Eaton Ltd., Regent House, The Broadway, Woking, Surrey GU21 5AP
Tel: Woking 71671
'Furasol' (Furaltadone 20%)
Paines & Byrne Ltd., Greenford
'Pancrex V'
Parke Davis & Co. Ltd., Warner-Lambert (UK) Ltd., Usk Road, Pontypool,
Gwent NP4 OYH
Tel: Pontypool (04955) 2468
'Abidec Drops' (Vits A,D,C,B, vitamins)
'Chloromycetin' preparations (Chloramphenicol)
'Kaogel' (Kaolin & pectin suspension)
'Vetalar' (Ketamine hydrochloride)
Pfizer Ltd., Sandwich, Kent CT13 9NJ
Tel: Sandwich (0304) 616161
'Terramycin' preparations (Oxytetracycline)
'Vibramycin' (doxycycline) Medical preparation.
Pharmavet Ltd., Industrial Estate, Riverview Road, Beverley, North Humberside
HU17 OLD
Multivitamin injection (Vitamins A, D_3, E and B vitamins)
A.H. Robins Company Ltd., Redkiln Way, Horsham, West Sussex RH13 5QP
Tel: Horsham (0403) 60361/4
'Dopram-V' (Doxapram hydrochloride)
Roche Products Ltd., P.O. Box 8, Welwyn Garden City, Herts. AL7 3AY
Tel: (07073) 28128
'Alcobon' (5-Fluorocystosine)
'Valium' injection (Diazepam) Medical preparation
Roussel Laboratories Ltd., Wembley Park, Middlesex HA9 0NF.
Tel: 01-903 1454
'Claforan' (Cefotaxime) medical preparation
Sinclair Pharmaceuticals Ltd., Borough Road, Godalming, Surrey GU7 2AB
Tel: (04868) 28222
'Ledclair' (Sodium calcium edetate) medical preparation
Smith Kline Animal Health Ltd., Cavendish Road, Stevenage, Hertfordshire
SG1 2EJ
Tel: (0438) 67881
'Vi-sorbin' (Vitamins B_{12}, B_6, iron and folic acid)
E.R. Squibb & Sons Ltd., Squibb House, 141/149 Staines Road, Hounslow
TW3 3JB
Tel: 01-572 7422
'Demavet' (Dimethyl sulphoxide)
'Fungizone' (Amphotericin injectable) ⎫
'Fungilin suspension' (Amphotericin)   ⎬   Medical preparation
'Nystan suspension' (Nystatin)   ⎭
'Mycostatin-20' (Nystatin powder)

'Ophthaine' (Proparacaine hydrochloride)
'Vionate' (Compound vitamin and mineral supplement)
Steinhard Ltd., 702-3 Tudor Estate, Abbey Road, London NW10 7UW
Tel: 01-965 0194
'Aluline' (Allopurinol)
Syntex Agribusiness, Syntex Pharmaceuticals Ltd., Syntex House, St. Ives Road,
Maidenhead, Berkshire SL6 1RD
Tel: (0628) 33191
'Tardak' (Delmadinone acetate)
Upjohn Ltd., Agricultural Veterinary Division, Fleming Way, Crawley, West
Sussex RH10 2NJ
Tel: Crawley (0293) 31133
'Kaobiotic suspension' (Kaolin sulphonamides neomycin)
'Kaopectate' (Kaolin suspension) Medical preparation
'Lincocin' preparations (Lincomycin hydrochloride)
'Neobiotic-P Aquadrops' (neomycin & methscopolamine)
'Panmycin Aquadrops' (Tetracycline hydrochloride)
'Promone-E' (Medroxyprogesterone)
Veterinary Drug Co. PLC, 129–135 Lawrence Street, York YO1 3EG
Tel: (0904) 412314
'Skin dressing derris 2%'
'Kaolin mixture B.P.C.'
'Atropine sulphate injection' B. Vet. C.
'Sodium calcium edentate veterinary' B. Vet. C.
'Piperazine'
'Pybuthrin dusting powder' (Piperony butoxide & pyrethrins)
The Wellcome Foundation Ltd., Veterinary & Agricultural Division, Crewe Hall,
Crewe, Cheshire CW1 1UB
Tel: (0270) 583151
'Ovigest elixir' (Protein digest & glucose)
'Septrin Paediatric suspension' (Trimethoprim & sulphamethoxazole) medical
preparation
'Tribrissen oral suspension' (Trimethoprim & sulphadiazin)
'Trivetrin injection' (Trimethoprim & sulfadoxine)
'Zyloric' (Allopurinol) Medical preparation
Willows Francis Veterinary, Division A.H. ROBINS, Redkiln Way, Horsham,
West Sussex RH13 5QP
Tel: (0403) 60361/4
'Auroid'
'Scorprin 120 capsules' (Trimethoprim & suphadiazine)
Winthrop Laboratories, Sterling Winthrop House, Surbiton, Surrey KT6 4PH
Tel: 01-399 5252
'Alevaire' (Tyloxapol)

13/Further Reading List

Arnall, L. & Keymer, I.F. (1975) *Bird Diseases*. Bailliere Tindall, London.

Cooper, J.E. (1978) *Veterinary Aspects of Captive Birds of Prey*. Standfast Press, Saul, Glos.

Cooper, J.E. & Eley J.T. (1979) *First Aid and Care of Wild Birds*. David & Charles, London.

Elkins, N. (1983) *Weather and Bird Behaviour*. T. A. D. Poyser Ltd., Carlton.

Fowler, M.E. (1978) *Zoo and Wild Animal Medicine*. W. B. Saunders Co., Philadelphia/London

Gordon, R. F. (1977) *Poultry Diseases*. Bailliére Tindall, London.

King, A.S. & McLelland, J. (1984) *Birds: Their Structure and Function*. Bailliére Tindall, London.

Mavrogordato, J. G. (1973) *A Hawk for the Bush*. 2nd edn Neville Spearman, London.

Petrak, M. L. (1969, 1982) *Diseases of Cage and Aviary Birds*, 1st and 2nd edns, Lea & Febiger, Philadelphia.

Ratcliffe, J. (1979) *Fly High, Run Free*. Chatto & Windus, London.

Steiner, C. V. & Davis R. B. (1981) *Caged Bird Medicine*. Iowa State University Press, Ames, Iowa.

Wallack J. D. & Boever, W. J. (1983) *Diseases of Exotic Animals; Medical and Surgical Management*. W. B. Saunders Co., Philadelphia/London.

Woodford, M. H. (1960) *A Manual of Falconry*. Adam & Charles Black, London.

14/References

Ahlers, W. (1977) Report on the use of bisolvon in small animal practice. *Kleintier-Praxis*, **15**, 50–53.

Altman, R. B. & Miller, M.S. (1979) The effect of Halothane and Ketamin anaesthesia on body temperature and electro-cardiographic changes of birds. *Proceedings of the American Association of Zoo Veterinarians*, Denver, Colorado, 61–62A.

Altman, R. B. (1980) Avian Anaesthesia. *The Compendium on Continuing Veterinary Education*, **2**, 38–42.

Altman, R. B. (1982) In: *Diseases of Cage and Aviary Birds* 2nd edn, (ed. M.L. Petrak), p. 369, Lea & Fibiger, Philadelphia.

Ar, A. & Rahn, H. (1977) Interdependence of gas conductance, incubation, length and weight of avian egg. In: "Respiratory Function in Birds, Adult and Embryonic", a satellite symposium of the *27th International Congress of Physiological Sciences, Paris 1977* (Ed. J. Piiper), pp. 227–236. Springer-Verlag, Berlin, Heileberg, New York.

Arañez, J. B. & Sanguin, C.S. (1955) Poulardization of native ducks. *Journal of the American Veterinary Medicine Association*, **127**, 314–317.

Aston, G. & Smith, H.G. (1984) *Psittacosis in Birds and Man*. The Unit for Veterinary Continuing Education, Vet 31, The Royal Veterinary College, London.

Bernier, G., Morin, M. & Marsolais, G. (1981) A generalised inclusion body disease in the budgerigar (*Melopsittacus undulatus*) caused by Papova-like agent. *Avian Diseases*, **23**, 1083–1093.

Berry, R. B. (1972) Reproduction by artificial insemination in captive American goshawks. *Journal of Wildlife Management*, **36**, 1283–1288.

Bird, D. M., Lague, P.C. & Buckland, R.B. (1976) Artificial insemination versus natural mating in captive American kestrels. *Canadian Journal of Zoology*, **54**, 1183–1191.

Blackmore, D. K. (1982) In: *Diseases of Cage and Aviary Birds* 2nd edn, (ed. M.L. Petrak), p. 484, Lea & Fibiger, Philadelphia.

Borland, E. D., Moryson, C.T., Smith, G.R. (1977) Avian botulism and the high prevalence of clostridium botulinum in the Norfolk broads. *Veterinary Record*, **100**, 106–109.

Bortch, A. & Vroege, C. (1972) Amputation of the wing under Rompun sedation and experimental sedation of the homing pigeon with Rompun. *Veterinary Review*, **(3/4)**, 275.

Böttcher, M. (1981) *Recent Advances in the Study of Raptor Diseases* (eds J.E. Cooper & A.G. Greenwood), pp. 89–93. Chiron Publications Ltd., Keighley, Yorks.

Boyd, L. L. (1978) Artificial Insemination of Falcons. *A Symposium of the Zoological Society of London*, **43**, 73–80.

Boyd, L. L. & Schwartz, C.H. (1983) Training imprinted semen donors. In: *Falcon Propagation, a Manual on Captive Breeding* (eds Weaver, J.D. & Cade, T.J.), p. 10. The Peregrine Fund, Inc. Ithaca, New York.

Brooks, N. G. (1982) Crop wall necrosis in a sparrowhawk. *Veterinary Record*, **3**, (22), 513.

Brown, L. (1976) *Birds of Prey: Their Biology and Ecology*, p. 117. Hamlyn, London.

Burnham, W., Walton, B.J. & Weaver, J.D. (1983) Management and maintenance. In: *Falcon Propagation, a Manual on Captive Breeding* (eds Weaver, J.D. & Cade, T.J.), p. 11. The Peregrine Fund, Inc. Ithaca, New York.

Bush, M. (1980) *Animal Laparascopy* (eds R. M. Harrison and D. E. Wildt), pp. 183–193. Williams and Wilkins, Baltimore/London.

Bush, M. (1981) Avian fracture repair using external fixation. In: *Recent Advances in the Study of Raptor Diseases* (eds J.E. Cooper and A.G. Greenwood), pp. 83–93. Chiron Publishers Ltd, Keighley, Yorks.

Bush, M., Montali, R.I., Novak, R.G. & James, F.A. (1976) The healing of avian fractures. A histological xeroradiographic study. *American Animal Hospital Association Journal*, **12**(6), 768–773.

Bush, M., Neal, L.A. & Custer, R.S. (1979) Preliminary pharmacokinetic studies of selected antibiotics in birds. *Proceedings of the American Association of Zoo Veterinarians* 45–47.

Bush, M., Locke, D., Neal, L.A. & Carpenter, J.W. (1981) Pharmacokinetics of Cephalin and Cephalexin in selected avian species. *American Journal of Veterinary Research*, **42**(6), 1014–1017.

Butler, E. J. & Laursen-Jones, A.P. (1977) Nutritional disorders. In: *Poultry Diseases* (ed. R.F. Gordon), p. 158. Bailliére Tindall, London.

Camburn, M. A. & Stead, C. (1966–1967) Anaesthesia of Wild Birds. *Proceedings of the Association of Veterinary Anaesthetists of Great Britain and Ireland*, **6**, 821.

Campbell, T. W. (1984) Diagnostic cytology in avian medicine. *Veterinary Clinics of North America* (ed. G.J. Harrison), **14**(2), 317–343.

Campbell, T. W. & Dein, F.J. (1984) Avian haematology—the basics. *Veterinary Clinics of North America* (ed. G.J. Harrison), **14**(2), 223–248.

Clubb, S. L. (1984) Therapeutics in avian medicine—flock vs. individual bird treatment regimens. *The Veterinary Clinics of North America* (ed. G. J. Harrison), **14**(2), 345–361.

Coffin, D. L. (1969) In: *Diseases of Parrots and Parrot-like Birds* (ed. the Duke of Bedford), p. 35. T.F.H. Publications, Inc., Hong Kong.

Coles, B. H. (1984a) Avian anaesthesia. *Veterinary Record*, **115**(12), 307.

Coles, B. H. (1984b) Some considerations when nursing birds in veterinary premises. *Journal of Small Animal Practice*, **25** (5), 275–288.

Cooke, S. W. (1984) Lead poisoning in cygnets. *Veterinary Record*, **114**(8), 203.

Cooper, J. E. (1970) The use of the hypnotic agent Methoxymol in birds of prey. *Veterinary Record*, **87**, 751–752.

Cooper, J. E. (1974) Metomidate anaesthesia of some birds of prey for laparotomy and sexing. *Veterinary Record*, **24**, 437–440.

Cooper, J. E. (1978) *Veterinary Aspects of Captive Birds of Prey*, pp. 21, 28. Standfast Press, Saul, Gloucestershire.

Cooper, J. E. (1983) In: *Sonderdruk aus Verhandlungs bericht des 25 internationalen Symposiums über die Erkrankungen* der Zootiere Wien Akademie verlag, Berlin, 61–65.

Cooper, J. E. & Redig, P. T. (1975) Unexpected reactions to the use of C.T. 1341 by red-tailed hawks. *Veterinary Record*, **97**, 352.

Cooper, M. E. (1979) *Wild bird hospitals and the law in first aid and care of wild birds.* (eds J.E. Cooper and J.T. Eley), pp. 15–30. David & Charles Ltd., London.

Cribb, P. H. & Haigh, J.C. (1977) Anaesthesia for avian species. *Veterinary Record*, **100**, 472–473.

Dawson, R. W. (1975) Avian physiology. *Annual Review of Physiology*, **37**, 441–465.

de Gruchy, P. H. (1983) Chlamydiosis in collared doves. *Veterinary Record*, **113** (14), 327.

Delius, J. D. (1966) Pentobarbitone Anaesthesia in the herring and black-backed gull. *Journal of Small Animal Practice*, **7**, 605–609.

Dunker, H. R. (1977) Development of the Avian Respiratory and Circulatory Systems; Respiratory function in birds, adult and embryonic. *Satellite Symposium of the 27th International Congress of Physiological Sciences, Paris 1977*, 267, Springer-verlag, Berlin.

Dunker, H. R. (1978) Coelom-Gliederung der Wirbeltiere-Funktionelle Aspekte. *Verh. Anat. Ges* **72**, 91–112.

Durant, A. J. (1926) Caecal abligation in fowls. *Veterinary Medicine*, **21**, 14–17.

Durant, A. J. (1930) Blackhead in turkeys, surgical control by caecal abligation. *Research Bulletin University of Missouri College of Agriculture* no. **133**.

Durant, A. J. (1953) Removal of the vocal cords of the fowl. *Journal of the American Veterinary Medical Association*, **122**, 14–17.

Elkins, N. (1983) *Weather and Bird Behaviour*, pp. 86–90. T. A. D. Poyser Ltd., Carlton.

Fedde, M. R. & Kuhlman, W.D. (1977) Intrapulmonary carbon-dioxide sensitive receptors: Amphibians to mammals. Respiratory function in birds, adult and embryonic. *Symposium of the 27th International Congress of Physiological Sciences, Paris* (ed. J. Piiper), pp. 30–50. Springer-verlag, Berlin.

Fiennes, T-W., R.N. (1969) Infectious diseases of bacterial origin. In: *Diseases of Cage and Aviary Birds* (ed. M.L. Petrak), pp. 361–369. Lea and Febiger, Philadelphia.

Forbes, N. A. (1984) Avian anaesthesia. *Veterinary Record*, **115**(6), 134.

Franchetti, D. R. & Klide, A.M. (1978) *Restraint and Anaesthesia in Zoo and Wild Animal Medicine* (ed. M.E. Fowler), p. 303, W. B. Saunders Co., Philadelphia.

Frith, H. J. (1959) Incubator birds. In: *Scientific American: Birds* (ed. B.W. Wilson), pp. 142–148. W. H. Freeman & Co., San Francisco.

Frith, C. W. & Greenwood, A.G. (1982) Treatment of aspergillosis in raptors. *Veterinary Record*, **111** (25/26), 584.

Galvin, C. E. (1978) Cage Bird Medicine. *Veterinary Clinics of North America*, **14**(2), p. 285.

Gass, H. (1979) *Kleintier-Praxis*, **34**, 393.

George, J. C. & Berger, A.J. (1966) *Avian Myology*. Academic Press, New York.

Gilbert, A. B. (1979) Female genital organs. In: *Form and Function in Birds* (Eds A.S. King & J. McLelland), **1**, p. 331. Academic Press Inc. (London) Ltd.

Gordon, R. F. & Jordan, F.T.W. (1977) Poultry Diseases, p. 219. Bailliere Tindall, London.

Graham-Jones, O. (1966) The clinical approach to tumours in cage birds III: Restraint and anaesthesia of small cage birds. *Journal of Small Animal Practice*, **7**, 231–239.

Green, C. J. (1979) Animal anaesthesia. In: *Laboratory Animal Handbooks 8*, pp. 126–128. Laboratory Animals Ltd., London.

Green, C. & Simpkin, S. (1984) Avian Anaesthesia. *The Veterinary Record*, **115**(7), 159.

Greenwood, A. G. & Barnett, K.C. (1980) The Investigation of the Visual Defects in Raptors. In: *Recent Advances in the Study of Raptor Diseases* (eds J.E. Cooper & A.G. Greenwood). Chiron Publications, Ltd., Keighley, Yorks.

Grier, J. W. (1973) Techniques and results of artificial insemination with golden eagles. *Raptor Research*, **7**, 1–12.

Grier, J. W., Berry, R.B. & Temple, S.A. (1972) Artificial insemination with imprinted raptors. *Journal of the American Falconers Association*, **11**, 45–55.

Haigh, J. C. (1980) Anaesthesia of raptorial birds. In: *Recent Advances in the Study of Raptor Diseases* (eds J.E. Cooper & A.G. Greenwood), 61–66. Chiron Publications Ltd., Keighley, Yorks.

Harcourt-Brown, N. H. (1978) Avian anaesthesia in general practice. *Journal of Small Animal Practice*, **19**, 573–582.

Harrison, G. J. (1984) New aspects of avian surgery. *Veterinary Clinics of North America*, **14**(2), 363–380.

Harrison, L. R. & Herron, A. J. (1984) Submission of diagnostic samples to a laboratory. *Veterinary Clinics of North America*, **14**(2), 165–172.

Hasholt, J. (1969) Diseases of the nervous system. In: *Diseases of Cage and Aviary Birds* (ed. M.L. Petrak). Lea and Febiger, Philadelphia.

Heck, R. W. & Konke, D. Incubation and Rearing. In: *Falcon Propagation, a Manual on Captive Breeding* (eds Weaver, J.D. & Cade, T.J.), p. 49. The Peregrine Fund, Inc., Ithaca, New York.

Hurrel, L. H. (1968) Wild raptor casualties. *Journal of Devon Trust*, **19**, 806–807.

Hill, K. J. & Noakes, D.E. (1964) Cyclopropane anaesthesia in the fowl. In: *Small Animal Anaesthesia: Proceeding of B.S.A.V.A./U.F.A.W. Symposium* (ed. O. Graham-Jones), p. 123–126. Pergamon, Oxford.

Ivins, G. K. (1975) Sex determination in raptorial birds—a study of chromatic bodies. *Journal of Zoo Animal Medicine*, **6**, 9–11.

Johnson, O. W. (1979) *Form and function in birds* (eds A.S. King & J. McLelland), Vol. 1, Academic Press, London.

Jojié, D. & Popovié, S. (1969) Artery vascularization of certain aerated bones of domestic hen and pigeon wings. *Acta Veterinaria* (Belgrade), **29**, 87—95.

Jones, C. G. (1980) Abnormal and maladaptive behaviour in captive raptors. In: *Recent advances in the study of raptor diseases.* (eds J.E. Cooper & A.G. Greenwood), Chiron Publications Ltd., Keighley, Yorks.

Jones, D. M. (1977) The sedation and anaesthesia of birds and reptiles. *Veterinary Record*, **101**, 340–342.

Jones, D. M. (1979) The nutrition of parrots: The husbandry and medicine of the parrot family. *Proceedings of B.V.Z.S./Parrot Society Meeting* (eds J.E. Cooper & A.G. Greenwood), p. 31. Regent's Park, London.

Jones, R. S. (1966) Halothane anaesthesia in turkeys. *British Journal of Anaesthesia*, **38**, 656–658.

Kendeigh, S. C. (1970) Energy requirements for the existence in relation to size of birds. *Condor*, **72**, 60.

Keymer, I. F. (1969) *Diseases of Cage and Aviary Birds*, 1st edn, (ed. M.L.

Petrak), p. 434. Lea & Febiger, Philadelphia.

King, A. S. & McLelland, J. (1975) (a and b) *Outlines of Avian Anatomy*, **46**, p. 6–7. Bailliere Tindall, London.

King, A. S. & McLelland, J. (1979) *Form and Function in Birds*. (eds A.S. King & J. McLelland), p. 74–79. Bailliere Tindall, London.

King, A. S. & McLelland, J. (1984) (a, b and c) *Birds: their structure and function*, pp. 64, 140–142, 311–312. Bailliere Tindall, London.

King, A. S. & Payne, D.C. (1964) Normal breathing and the effects of posture in *Gallus domesticus*. *Journal of Physiology*, **174**, 340–347.

Kirkwood, J. F. (1981) Recent advances in the study of raptor diseases. In: *Proceedings of the International Symposium on Diseases of Birds of Prey* (eds J.E. Cooper & A.G. Greenwood), pp. 153–157, Chiron Publications Ltd., Keighley, Yorks.

Klide, A. M. (1973) Avian anaesthesia. *Veterinary Clinics of North America*, **3**(2), 175–186.

Kock, M. (1983) Sexing birds. *Veterinary Record*, **112**(19), 463.

Kovách, A. G. B. & Szász, E. (1968) Survival of pigeons after graded haemorrhage. *Acta Physiologica*, **34**(301).

Kovách, A. G. B., Szász, E. & Pilmayer, N. (1969) The mortality of various avian and mammalian species following blood loss. *Acta. P. N. Acad. Sci.* 35–109.

Lack, D. (1975) *The life of the robin*, 4th ed. H. F. and G. Witherby, London.

Lasiewski, R. C. & Dawson, L.R. (1967) A re-examination of the relation between standard metabolic rate and bodyweight of birds. *Condor*, **69**, 13–23.

Lawrence, K. (1983) Treatment of aspergillosis in raptors. *Veterinary Record*, **112**(4), 80.

Lawrence, K. (1983) Efficacy of fenbendazole against nematodes of captive birds. *Veterinary Record*, **112**(18), 433–434.

Lawton, P. C. (1984) Avian anaesthesia. *Veterinary Record*, **115**(3), 71.

Levinger, I. M., Kedem, J. & Abram, M. (1973) A new anaesthetic-sedative preparation for birds. *British Veterinary Journal*, **129**, 296–300.

Lorenz, K. (1935) Companions as factors in the bird's environment. In: *Studies in Animals and Human Behaviour* (1970 edn, trans. R. Martin), Vol. 1. Methuen, London.

Lorenz, K. (1937) The companions in the bird's world. *Auk*, **54**, 245–273.

Lorenz, K. (1965) Die "Erfindung" von Flugmaschen in der Evolution der Wirbeltiere. In: *Darwin hat recht gesehen*. Neske verlag.

McKeever, K. (1979) *Care and Rehabilitation of Injured Owls*, pp. 24–25, 92, 94. W.F. Rannie, Lincoln, Ontario, Canada.

McMillan, M. C. (1982) (a, b and c) *Diseases of Cage and Aviary Birds*, 2nd edn, (ed. M.L. Petrak), pp. 330, 340, 359. Lea and Febiger, Philadelphia.

Mandelker, L. (1972) Ketamine hydrochloride as an anaesthetic for parakeets. *Veterinary Medicine/Small Animal Clinician*, **67**, 55–56.

Mandelker, L. (1973) A Toxicity Study of Ketamine HCL in Parakeets. *Veterinary Medicine/Small Animal Clinician*, **68**, 487–489.

Mangilgi, G. (1971) Unilateral patagiectomy: A new method of preventing flight in captive birds. In: *International Zoo Year Book XI*, pp. 252–254.

Marley, E. & Payne, J.P. (1964) Halothane anaesthesia in the fowl. In: *Small animal anaesthesia proceedings of a B.S.A.V.A./U.F.A.W. Symposium* (ed. O.

Graham-Jones), p. 127. Pergamon, Oxford.

Mavrogordato, J. G. (1973) *A Hawk for the Bush*, 2nd edn, Neville Spearman, London.

Murdock, H. R. & Lewis, J.O.D. (1964) A simple method for obtaining blood from ducks. *Proceedings of the Society for Experimental Biology and Medicine*, **116**, 51–52.

Murrell, L. R. (1975–76) A practical method of determining bird sex by chromosome analysis. *Annual Proceedings of the American Association of Zoological Parks and Aquariums*, 87–90.

Needham, J. R. (1981) Bacterial flora of birds of prey. In: *Recent Advances in the Study of Raptor Diseases* (eds J.E. Cooper and A.G. Greenwood), pp. 3–9. Chiron Publishers Ltd., Keighley, Yorks.

Newton, I. (1979) *Population ecology of raptors*. T. A. D. Poyser Ltd., p. 81–94.

Olney, P. J. S. (1958/9) *Wild Fowl Trust Report II*, p. 154. Slimbridge, Glos.

Pass, D. A. & Perry, R.A. (1984) The pathology of psittacine beak and feather disease. *Australian Veterinary Journal*, **61**(3), pp. 69–74.

Peakall, D. B. (1970) Pesticides and reproduction of birds. In: *Scientific American: Birds* (ed. B.W. Wilson), pp. 255–261. W. H. Freeman and Company, San Francisco.

Perrins, C. M. (1979) *British Tits*, pp. 160, 260–261. Collins, London.

Philip, H.R.H. Prince (1984) *Address to General Assembly of the International Union for Conservation of Nature and Natural Resources*. Madrid.

Rahn, H., Ar, A. & Pagenelli, C.V. (1979) How birds breathe. In: *Scientific American: Birds* (ed. B.W. Wilson), pp. 208–217. W. H. Freeman and Company, San Francisco.

Redig, P. T. (1978) Raptor rehabilitation: diagnosis, prognosis and moral issues. *Conference on Bird of Prey Management Techniques, Oxford*. (ed. T.A. Greer).

Redig, P. T. (1979) *First and and care of wild birds* (eds. J.E. Cooper & J.T. Eley). David & Charles, Newton Abbot.

Redig, P. T. (1981) Aspergillosis in raptors. In: *Recent Advances in the Study of Raptor Diseases* (eds J.E. Cooper & A.G. Greenwood), pp. 117–122. Chiron Publications Ltd., Keighley, Yorks.

Redig, P. T. (1983) Anaesthesia for raptors. *Raptor Research & Rehabilitation Program*, newsletter 4, 9–10.

Redig, P. T. & Duke, G.E. (1976) Intravenously administered ketamine and diazepam for anaesthesia of raptors. *Journal of the American Veterinary Medical Association*, **169**, 886–888.

Reece, R. L. (1982) Observations on the accidental poisoning of birds by organophosphate insecticides and other toxic substances. *Veterinary Record*, **111**(20), 453.

Reiser, M. H. & Temple, S.A. (1980) Effects of chronic lead ingestion on birds of prey. In: *Recent Advances in the Study of Raptor Diseases* (eds J.E. Cooper & A.G. Greenwood), pp. 21–25. Chiron Publications Ltd., Keighley, Yorks.

Richards, J. R. (1980) Current concepts in the metabolic responses to injury, infection and starvation. *Proceedings of the Nutrition Society*, **39**, 113.

Richardson, J. D. (1984) Avian anaesthesia. *Veterinary Record*, **115**(7), 154.

Robinson, P. (1975) Unilateral patagiectomy. A technique for deflighting large birds. *Veterinary Medicine/Small Animal Clinician*, **70**(2), 143.

Rosskopf, W. J. & Woerpel, R.W. (1982) Abdominal surgery in pet birds.

Modern Veterinary Practice, **63**(2), 889–890.

Rosskopf, W. J., Woerpel, R.W. & Pitts, B.J. (1983) Surgical repair of a chronic cloacal prolapse in a greater sulphur crested cockatoo (*Cacatua galerita*). *Veterinary Medicine/Small Animal Clinician*, **78**(5), 719–724.

Samour, J. H., Jones, D.M., Knight, J.A. & Howlett, J.C. (1984) Comparative studies of the use of some injectable anaesthetic agents in birds. *Veterinary Record*, **115**(1), 6–11.

Schlotthauer, C. F., Essex, H.E. & Mann, F.C. (1933) Caecal occlusion in the prevention of Blackhead (enterohepatitis) in turkeys. *Journal of the American Veterinary Medical Association*, **83**, 218.

Scott, D. C. (1968) Intramedullary fixation of a fractured humerus in a wild owl. *Canadian Veterinary Journal*, **9**, 98–99.

Secord, A. C. (1958) Fractures in birds repaired with the Jonas splint. *Veterinary Medicine*, **53**, 655–656.

Small, E. (1969) In: *Diseases of Cage and Aviary Birds*, 1st edn, (Ed. M.L. Petrak), p. 354, Lea & Febiger, Philadelphia.

Smith, G. A. (1979) Parrot disease as encountered in a veterinary practice. In: *"The Husbandry and Medicine of the Parrot Family"—the proceedings of a B.V.Z.S./Parrot Society meeting, Regent's Park, London*. (eds A.G. Greenwood & J.E. Cooper).

Smith, G. A. (1982) *Magazine of the Parrot Society*, **16**(11), 340.

Steiner, C. V. & Davis, R.B. (1981) *Caged Bird Medicine*, p. 136. Iowa State University Press, Ames, Iowa.

Stettenheim, P. (1972) The integument of birds. In: *Avian Biology, Vol. II* (eds Farner, King & Parks), 7. Academic Press, New York/London.

Stunkard, J. A. & Miller, J.C. (1974) An Outline Guide to General Anaesthesia in Exotic Species. *Veterinary Medicine/Small Animal Clinician*, **69**: 1181–1186.

Sykes, A. H. (1964) Some aspects of anaesthesia in the adult fowl in *Small Animal Anaesthesia—Proceedings of a B.S.A.V.A./U.F.A.W. Symposium, London, 1963* (ed. O. Graham-Jones), pp. 117–121. Pergamon, Oxford.

Temple, S. A. (1972) Artificial insemination with imprinted birds of prey. *Nature*, **237**, 287–288.

Tiemeier, O. W. (1941) Repairing bone injuries. *Auk*, **58**, 350–359.

Von Becker, E. (1974) Schnabelschienung bel Afrikanischen Hornraben Praktische *tieräkzt*, **55**(9), 492–494.

Wallack, J. D. & Boever, W.J. (1983) *Diseases of Exotic Animals: Medical and Surgical Management*. W. B. Saunders Co., Philadelphia.

Weaver, J. D. (1983) Artificial insemination. In: *Falcon Propagation, a Manual on Captive Breeding*. (eds Weaver, J.D. & Cade, T.J.), pp. 19–23. The Peregrine Fund, Inc., Ithaca, New York.

Wilgus, H. S. (1960) Reserpine for tranquillising geese. *The 2nd Conference on the use of Reserpine in Poultry Production*. The Institute of Agriculture, Minnesota, St. Paul, Minnesota, 54–56.

Wilkinson, J. S. (1984) A.I. Work in France. *Journal of the Welsh Hawking Club*, 9–13.

Woerpel, R. W. & Rosskopf, W.J. (1984) Clinical experience with avian laboratory diagnostics. In: Symposium on caged bird medicine. *The Veterinary Clinics of North America* **14**(2), 249–286.

Zenobe, R. D. & Egger, E.L. (1980) Use of colopexy to correct eversion of the cloacal mucosa in a mynah bird. *Veterinary Medicine/Small Animal Clinician*, **79**(9), 1427–1428.

Index

Page references in *italics* refer to figures or tables.